PRAISE FOR

Connected Fates, Separate Destinies

'With *Connected Fates, Separate Destinies*, Marine provides
all of us with a map to help orient ourselves
within the web of our origin stories.'

— Ruby Warrington, author of *Sober Curious*

'*Connected Fates, Separate Destinies* is a powerful, potent, and
magical book that will help you recognize the hidden patterns
in your life that make the biggest difference, so you can clear
them once and for all and live a life of greater peace and
acceptance. I highly recommend this book for
every single person on the planet.'

— Sahara Rose, bestselling author of *Discover Your Dharma*

'Marine Sélénée offers enlightened wisdom and practical tools
to make peace with your past and create your dream future,
through Family Constellations therapy. Now, more than ever,
we all need to fall madly in love with ourselves and after
reading this book, you will be well on your way.'

— Sah D'Simone, author of *Spiritually Sassy*
and *5-Minute Daily Meditations*

'Marine Sélénée has a true gift. *Connected Fates, Separate Destinies* gracefully guides you to your highest source of healing, which is found when you seek within. This book provides a mirror to seeing your highest self, and learning to honor your lineage through love, care, and reverence.'

— Rosie Acosta, author, yoga and meditation teacher, and host of the *Radically Loved* podcast

'Marine offers a fascinating picture of family constellations and its hidden energetic structures within the family system. In short, she explains that whatever we reject is what we repeat. This book is an offering to your soul that will compel you to rewrite your story, accept your family, and break the cycle once and for all. As Marine's client and friend, I enthusiastically endorse her teachings and guidance. Pay attention to this book because there is so much to learn here.'

— Bee Bosnak, spiritual teacher and business mentor

Connected Fates, Separate Destinies

Connected Fates, Separate Destinies

USING FAMILY CONSTELLATIONS THERAPY TO RECOVER FROM INHERITED STORIES AND TRAUMA

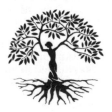

MARINE SÉLÉNÉE

HAY HOUSE

Carlsbad, California • New York City
London • Sydney • New Delhi

Published in the United Kingdom by:
Hay House UK Ltd, The Sixth Floor, Watson House,
54 Baker Street, London W1U 7BU
Tel: +44 (0)20 3927 7290; Fax: +44 (0)20 3927 7291; www.hayhouse.co.uk

Published in the United States of America by:
Hay House Inc., PO Box 5100, Carlsbad, CA 92018-5100
Tel: (1) 760 431 7695 or (800) 654 5126
Fax: (1) 760 431 6948 or (800) 650 5115; www.hayhouse.com

Published in Australia by:
Hay House Australia Ltd, 18/36 Ralph St, Alexandria NSW 2015
Tel: (61) 2 9669 4299; Fax: (61) 2 9669 4144; www.hayhouse.com.au

Published in India by:
Hay House Publishers India, Muskaan Complex, Plot No.3, B-2,
Vasant Kunj, New Delhi 110 070
Tel: (91) 11 4176 1620; Fax: (91) 11 4176 1630; www.hayhouse.co.in

Text © Marine Sélénée, 2021

Project editor: Melody Guy • *Indexer:* J S Editorial, LLC
Cover design: Howie Severson • *Interior design:* Bryn Starr Best
Author Photo: Camila Gutiérrez

A catalogue record for this book is available from the British Library.

Tradepaper ISBN: 978-1-78817-817-4
E-book ISBN: 978-1-4019-6206-7
Audiobook ISBN: 978-1-4019-6207-4

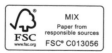

MIX
Paper from
responsible sources
FSC
www.fsc.org   FSC® C013056

Printed and bound in Great Britain by
TJ Books Limited, Padstow, Cornwall

TO THE MEN OF MY LIFE

TO MEHDI

Contents

Foreword xi

Introduction: Happiness Is an Achievement of the Soul xvii

Chapter 1:   Origin Stories. 1

Chapter 2:   Belonging, Order, and Entanglement. 39

Chapter 3:   The Only Right Parents. 61

Chapter 4:   Enlightened Love 91

Chapter 5:   Yes, Yes, Yes 125

Chapter 6:   From Fragmentation to Wholeness. 151

Conclusion: Healing Is an Act of Faith 173

Reading List 181

Endnotes 182

Index 183

Acknowledgments 193

About the Author 197

Foreword

In another life I might have been either a psychologist or an anthropologist. I've always been fascinated by people and what makes them tick; why are we the way we are? As a kid, I looked for the answer to this question in novels. As a teenager, I sought it out on the loved-up dance floors of the early rave scene. In my career as a magazine journalist, I wrote about social trends and conducted probing interviews in which I tried to decipher the inner state of A-list celebrities by the way they sipped their coffee. When I subsequently found astrology, I finally had a language to describe the numinous, unseen, and undefinable parts of the human experience. All of which coalesces for me in Family Constellations therapy—a practice which has also helped me understand my need to understand.

I experienced my first constellation with Marine Sélénée in the spring of 2014. I had moved to New York from the U.K. two years prior, a move that had sparked a period of feverish soul-searching. Cut adrift from my motherland and with 3,500 miles separating me from my family of origin, I found myself looking back across the Atlantic with a fresh perspective on where I had come from. This coincided with me deciding to cut alcohol out of my life, and as the boozy fog of my twenties and early thirties began to lift, more questions came into focus: Why had I felt the pull to America? Why did I feel more "me" the farther I was from my family? Why had I never wanted to have kids of my own? And why, despite having worked so hard to achieve all the external markers of a "successful" life, was my own inner resting state one of anxiety and melancholy?

That rainy afternoon in SoHo, and over subsequent sessions with Marine, I discovered some new answers. When I pressed the buzzer to her apartment, my heart a hummingbird in my chest, I had no idea what to expect. At the time, I was busy establishing my "Now Age" lifestyle platform, The Numinous, and I had thrown myself headfirst into my research; I was the awkward Brit at the healing circle, learning one anguished sob at a time that it was okay to cry in front of a room full of strangers. I'd recently even attended my first "spirit séance," where the psychic medium leading the session had guided us to receive our own messages from "the other side." How would my afternoon with Marine measure up?

Inside, I was introduced to the two other women who would be participating in the constellation. I don't remember if I ever learned their names. Then, one by one, Marine carefully conducted our individual family dramas. When it was my turn, it was like time and space fell away as the edges of my vision blurred to nothingness. Marine invited the woman representing my "mother" to turn and face me. In that moment, I saw myself *as my mother's mother*, the grandmother I had never known, while the face of the woman in front of me morphed into that of my mum as a little girl: *my child*. A wave of grief churned through me, and I sobbed again as my body was flooded with our mutual loss: three generations of women with no motherland to ground us, lost and all at sea.

The experience was both healing and deeply trippy, like therapy on LSD, and over the following two years my sessions with Marine would bring similarly profound moments of insight. Realizations that I might have been able to come to an intellectual understanding of in talk therapy, but which now landed in my body with such shocking clarity there was no mistaking the imprint that my origin story had left on me. It was like the lights going on in a previously dark and scary basement, the dust sheets lifted from family secrets I could now see I had spent my whole life stumbling over. If I had always wanted to know why we are the way we are, then diving deep into the energy field of my ancestral lineage meant the clues were finally starting to add up.

And now, with *Connected Fates, Separate Destinies*, Marine provides all of us with a map to help orient ourselves within the web of our origin stories. My early interactions with Family Constellations therapy needed no further explanation; I got exactly what I needed from my work with Marine, and I didn't need to know how or why it had "worked." All that mattered was that I had been able to unravel the knotted threads of my family history, the better to disentangle myself from the past and actually live the life that my parents had handed down to me. But healing is a forever work in progress, and having access to the full philosophy behind the practice has been similarly revelatory.

For example, it was only a few months before I engaged with the work in this book that I discovered that I am the third "sister" on my father's side to seek a new life, severed from my immediate family, in the United States. My aunt Sarah, who I idolized and who passed the week before I sat down to write this foreword, had moved to California at age 20. But what I didn't know was that I also had a *great* aunt Ursula. She, too, had become a U.S. citizen and, like me, had never become a mother—following instead a queer life path that, in the words of my father, had seen her "expunged" from the family history. Could it be that both Sarah and myself had been "recruited" by the family system to reinstate Ursula's legacy? As Marine writes: "By recognizing every member of the system (granting them belonging) and allowing them their rightful place (restoring order), you release any unconscious loyalties you may have been carrying." Reading this, I found myself wondering: *How much of my restless sense of unbelonging had never actually belonged to me?*

Panning out, we might ask ourselves: How much of *our* unbelonging, how much of our lonely disconnectedness, and how much unprocessed pain and grief are we carrying on behalf of the ancestors who came before us? Ancestors who suffered so much within the varying systems of oppression that defined the era of colonialism. Marine's book is also coming at a time when the collective wounding of our ancestors is front and center in the collective consciousness, a time of reckoning with the legacy of our violent and extractive shared history. Healing these lesions means equipping ourselves with tools and practices for honoring what has been, and for processing what residual traumas have been passed down to us at the cellular level—and by making Family Constellations theory accessible to all, *Connected Fates, Separate Destinies* is offering exactly that.

Perhaps the most important teaching of all, which Marine drives home with a firm yet loving hand throughout her book, is that the past can never be undone. Our family will always be our family; our history, our history. Whatever tragedies and injustices have befallen those who came before us, it is not our job or our responsibility to continue to suffer on their behalf. "We cannot rectify the past; we can only acknowledge it and then attempt to break its patterns, beginning with ourselves," she writes, while reminding us to embody the mantra: "I guess this is the way it was meant to be, because it is the only way it was."

This is where her work dovetails with mine in the sober curious movement. In sobriety circles, the process of "recovery" is used to describe the journey of uncovering your own inner nature—the journey back to the "self" that was there all along, before the drink and the drugs (or the work, the food, and the relationship dramas) got layered on top like nullifying Band-Aids. A self that was born happy and whole, and which has often become entangled in unconscious agreements to shoulder the burden of our ancestors' pain in the misguided belief that if only we can make things right on their behalf, then order will be restored, and the equilibrium of our lineage reinstated. In many cases, sobriety is what creates the clarity for unacknowledged wounds to surface, recovery (in the words of the famous prayer) then lying in our ability to find "the serenity to accept the things we cannot change and the courage to change the things we can."

It's one thing to be able to understand the shape of our emotional inheritance, to be able to discern its weight and to navigate the space that it takes up in our lives. When the healing happens is when we're able to take conscious actions to break the patterns of our lineage—to free ourselves first and foremost, but also on behalf of those who came before and of the generations to come. *Connected Fates, Separate Destinies* shows us how to do just that.

Ruby Warrington
Brooklyn, NY

Introduction

Happiness Is an Achievement of the Soul

Like so many of my clients in my Family Constellations practice, as well as my friends and family, I spent years—*a lot* of years—in therapy. For most of my twenties, I was deeply unfulfilled, but the *why* remained murky at best, a target I shot at in darkness, or at the least, twilight. In therapy, I talked about my parents' divorce; my father's estrangement from the family; my own reckless and unfulfilling marriage, then subsequent divorce; and, eventually, being a stranger in a strange land, otherwise known as being French in America. And though the experience held value, my progress toward the person I hoped to be—and the life I wanted for myself—was painstakingly slow. The fact that the needle moved grudgingly in that time, if at all, seemed normal to me; I'd known *lots* of people in lifelong therapy. That was just how it worked, right? Still, I found myself seeking more—a bigger shift. *The* big shift.

Then, in 2012, an unexpected encounter radically altered not only my perception of self but of my place in the world, and of the world around me. In a single day, I received the kind of profound insights and emotional resolutions that had previously come only after three years of EMDR (eye movement desensitization and reprocessing) therapy, a type of psychotherapy designed to treat trauma through safe exposure to triggering memories. At the time, I was living in Miami and practicing meditation seriously. Okay, I was *struggling* with meditation seriously (while partying seriously . . . I was working in PR, after all). But my meditation teacher, Michelle Blechner, was one of the wisest women I'd met in my life, so I attempted to power through, eager to absorb some of her clarity and grace. Over tea one unremarkable afternoon, Michelle recounted to me her recent trip to New York City. She was incredibly excited about a new-to-her discovery she had made there, a therapeutic method called Family Constellations. She asked me if I wanted to attend a Family Constellations workshop with her later that week; she had already invited a facilitator, Natalie Berthold, to come lead one at her home.

I had no real idea what Family Constellations was, only that it took place in a group and that Michelle said it was too experiential to really describe. Her enthusiasm for it was so infectious, though, that she got my full attention. I was an old pro at talking about my family in therapy. How different could this be? As it turns out, *really* different. Really, really different. My life was about to change forever. Within two years, I myself would be a certified Family Constellations therapist, with my own thriving practice in New York City.

But just what is Family Constellations, anyway? And why should you care?

Though it's more of a philosophy than a therapy (more on that in a bit), it's fair to say that Family Constellations is a *therapeutic approach* that considers individuals as part of a greater transgenerational whole called a "family system," rather than as lone actors. Designed to reveal the hidden dynamics that underlie family systems, Family Constellations illuminates how the lives of those who've come before us—including those we've never known—actively shape our lives today, through the legacy of inherited traumas, in ways that are not likely to be clear to us.

So rather than focus on childhood conflicts, as much of traditional therapy does, it focuses instead on how historical events such as the loss of a parent, sibling, or child; the experience of war; or a sexual assault, to name just a few, reverberate through the family system, exerting a powerful, though often unrecognized, force on later generations. In the wake of such *intergenerational trauma*, Family Constellations posits, many of us become "entangled" with the unhappiness of those who came before us—unconsciously adopting destructive familial patterns of anxiety, depression, failure, and even illness and addiction in an attempt to "redo" the past and "fix" our families.

These hidden dynamics are made visible through the practice of an exercise called a "constellation." A constellation is done in a group setting or in a one-on-one meeting (in person or remotely) with a facilitator. First, a client expresses an issue he or she wants to work on, then intuitively organizes the group members (or symbolic stand-ins such as figurines) in relation to each other in the center of the room. After everyone is placed, the constellation—the pattern created by the group members' placement in relation to each other, like the stars in the night sky—emerges, reflecting the nature of the family system, uncovering entanglements through the literal positioning of the representatives.

Being able to perceive that we are part of a *system* shifts our focus from the actions of individuals to the dynamics of the family. When we make this shift, we experience a clarity of perception both radical and liberating. Family Constellations work builds the muscle of disinterested observation, where we go from biased subjects to neutral observers. Family Constellations requires that we switch from a fixation on "who harmed me" to the more dispassionate frame "how does this event reflect a harmful pattern in my family system." Doing so helps us escape the existing narratives that imprison us in unhealthy behaviors and relationships. People who don't want to be responsible for their lives and, thus, stay stuck in their stories—i.e., cling to blame—are not great candidates for Family Constellations.

Bert Hellinger, the German psychotherapist who developed Family Constellations, described this requirement of disinterested observation, of shifting our vision from the individual to the system, as the foundation of a "phenomenological" methodology of healing. As he wrote, "Phenomenology is a philosophical approach. For me, it means subjecting myself [as therapist] to larger contexts and connections, without needing to understand them. I accept them without any intention of helping or proving anything."

In many ways, it is not surprising that Family Constellations emerged in the decades after postwar Germany's confrontation with its recent and blood-soaked history—a history so dehumanizing that it could make conventional "understanding" impossible. Hellinger himself resisted Nazism (his refusal to join the Hitler Youth resulted in him being labeled a "suspected enemy of the state") but was eventually conscripted into the regular German Army, where he saw combat on the Western Front, before being captured by the Allies. Postwar, Hellinger entered the Catholic religious order of the Jesuits, studying philosophy and theology at university as part of his ordination.

Hellinger began forming his philosophy of Family Constellations in the early 1950s, while serving as a Jesuit priest on a mission in South Africa, where he lived for 16 years. The years he spent there working with and learning from the Zulu peoples and culture—in particular the Zulu worldview, *ubuntu*, often translated as "I am because we are"—came to shape his own worldview profoundly. Simultaneously, he developed an interest in phenomenology—within psychology, the study of subjective experience—through a series of interracial, ecumenical trainings in group dynamics led by Anglican clergy. Coming to grips with the realization that people were more important to him than abstracted ideals, Hellinger left the priesthood in the late 1960s and went to Vienna, where he trained in and practiced classical psychoanalysis. In a country struggling to come to terms with the genocide it had perpetrated on its own citizens—citizens who had been "otherized" and stripped of their humanity based on their ethnic-religious identity—Hellinger intuitively answered the call of those seeking tools not only for healing intergenerational trauma but also for preventing its repetition.

The beauty of the Family Constellations approach is that it empowers us to heal the root cause of our pain, rather than just treat the symptoms. Once a dynamic is revealed, we can break its patterns and disentangle ourselves from intergenerational trauma, no longer trying to control that which cannot be controlled: the past. In doing so, we also acknowledge our ancestors' place in that system and affirm their right to belong, honoring their fate and leaving their destinies at their feet, where they belong, unraveling the binding threads of entanglement. When we are no longer expending our energy trying to redo the past, however unwittingly, we are free to set down the burden of living in service to those who came before us and to step forward into a future of our own making. We are free to reclaim our destiny. Family Constellations reminds us: *You are not your conflict.* Understanding your past, owning your present, creating your future—that is the essence of Family Constellations.

Family Constellations offers a radical new perspective, one that affords us a broad, systemic view that decenters the self in favor of a "networked" way of seeing—that is, a way of seeing that highlights our interconnection, with our families and with each other. It reveals the role we play in a larger system, and the ways in which our traumas and our battles are part of an inherited legacy. And it reminds us that though our fates (that hand of cards we are each dealt by the universe) are connected to those of our ancestors, our destinies (the way we play them) are separate. They are our own.

Through understanding our family members' histories and pasts we make peace with ourselves. We see that the key to healing our wounds lives less in our own life experiences and more in those of our parents, grandparents, and even great-grandparents. Through recognizing the struggles of our ancestors, we acknowledge that our pains are a collective wound that never healed. This integration adds a new dimension to the healing process, creating a pathway for deep repair. We emerge feeling lighter, whole, like more genuine versions of ourselves. Like traditional therapy, Family Constellations turns toward the past. Rather than endlessly revisiting it, however, Family Constellations works to free you from its grasp, allowing you to leave behind the heavy weight of your old stories in order to write new ones—to fully be the author of your own life, on the path of your highest destiny.

There were only four people at my first constellation, that far-away afternoon in 2012. It was a small and private group, which was a relief. I was nervous—I didn't know what to expect or how to act. The serenity and professionalism of the facilitator, Natalie, quickly soothed my anxiety. Sitting in a small circle in Michelle's living room, we began. Natalie asked what issue I wanted to work on. I said I wanted to attract the love of my life and figure out why he had not yet arrived (I was not-so-newly divorced and still caught up in an on-again, off-again affair with my ex-husband, compelled by the drama of our disastrous marriage).

After asking a few more questions regarding my family history and dynamics, Natalie proposed I choose one person to represent my mother and another person to represent my father. I guided my "mother" to the center of the room, where she stood with a remarkably straight spine, somehow occupying more space than should have been possible. I seated my "father" next to her (Charlie, Michelle's husband, represented my father; he was 90 at the time and in the early stages of dementia). Charlie was one of the sweetest men I have ever met, and though his short-term memory was shot, he was an amazing representative. When Charlie took his place as my father, I was able to see my father's soul through his eyes. This deep connection was unexpected. How could Charlie represent my dad so well without even knowing him or his background? How had he embodied his energy so eerily? I was speechless.

Natalie then added a third representative to the group, my longed-for "man." She (the gender of the representative is of no importance in Family Constellations) went straight to the center of the room, without hesitation. We were in a small living room—the coffee table had been pushed aside to facilitate the constellation—and I felt an overwhelming impulse to get away. As my "man" was between me and the door, I moved to the corner and turned to face the wall. I literally did not want to be close with my partner. Dread crawled over my skin.

My first Family Constellations session lasted 40 minutes. At first, I let myself simply feel and be, but I began to resist as a truth crystallized that I did not want to see: I was afraid of love, and therefore, my future partner. My "father's" seated position reflected the power imbalance in my parents' dynamic: my father's passivity and my mother's strength. In a constellation, when a representative sits, they are often telling us that they are weak—they are tired, unable to stand. My mother's strength was dominating in a way that seemed to take up more room than was required.

Like my mother, I had married a weak man (though his weakness manifested itself in violence and possessiveness) and attempted to fix him. In fact, I'd had a series of weak boyfriends, one after the other. What my parents did not get right, I would. Of course, this did not work—I could not redo my mother and father's marriage and repair our family system. Being a nursemaid could not make me happy, and more than that, I was not able to live my destiny fully while attempting to carry my parents'. Yet when my man appeared—strong and purposeful, with no need of nursing—I had not only run away but turned my back on him, unable to look him in the face. I wasn't ready for a partnership of equals, despite my professed desire. I didn't want another injured lover, but I didn't know another way of being in relationship.

As my resistance to acknowledging the dynamic faltered, however, and I accepted what was, I began to feel immense relief and a strange optimism I had not experienced before. Suddenly, the urgency I felt around finding the love of my life, and the negative thoughts that accompanied it, had dissipated. The constellation had shown me that my heart was broken, and I needed to repair it before seeking out further relationships. I had to work on myself and heal my past before I could find love. This solution was my responsibility alone, and it gave me strength to keep going.

The power of that revelation and the sense of freedom—and power—I derived from it remained. I kept expecting it to dissolve, but there it was, resolute and steadfast, for days, then weeks, then months, until it was part of me. Meanwhile, I stopped expecting anything from my ex-husband after the constellation and was at peace with the situation. I had never experienced such a palpable and concrete shift before then.

I guess you could say I became a bit obsessed with Family Constellations. For a year and a half after that experience, I did constellations almost weekly, not only to address the thorny knots of my own emotional well-being but acting as a representative in others' constellations. The power, beauty, vulnerability, and deep humanity I witnessed and experienced filled me with not only profound gratitude but curiosity. The positive changes and growth not only in myself but also in others were undeniable.

Increasingly, I no longer wanted to work in publicity. I felt a calling to serve others, to become a facilitator in my own right. My first step was completing a formal training in Miami with Mark Wolynn, director of the Family Constellation Institute, the Inherited Trauma Institute, and co-founder of the Bert Hellinger Institute (Northern California), author of *It Didn't Start With You: How Inherited Family Trauma Shapes Who We Are and How to End the Cycle*, and one of the most renowned experts on and leaders in Family Constellations. Step two? Quitting my job entirely and taking a leap of faith: I left Miami and headed for New York to deepen my Family Constellations education—and I never looked back.

In New York, I found my home. I trained with the *other* most renowned Family Constellations therapist: Suzi Tucker, co-founder of the Bert Hellinger Institute (New York) and editor in chief of Zeig, Tucker & Theisen, Publishers, the primary English-language publishers of the work of Bert Hellinger. There, safe in the field, under the care of Suzi's fierce heart and strong but gentle guidance, I was finally able to acknowledge and consent to the reality of my most painful—and secret—burden: the sexual assault I had suffered at 13, about which I had told only one person: my therapist, though I had resisted addressing it.

Before Family Constellations, I had done my best to never think about the assault, though the trauma always caught up with me, as much as I tried to run from it. I compartmentalized the rape as something random that had happened to me, that was separate from my family and my issues with them. Through Family Constellations, I was able to reconcile the seemingly incongruous parts of my identity, integrating the assault into my life—seeing it clearly, finally, as part of a pattern of trauma that haunted my family—and, joyfully, I was also able to release the potent symptoms of the trauma, especially my barely suppressed and uncontrollable rage. I was able to reconcile with my past and restore peace to my relationship with the present, and to myself. Most critically, I was able to reconcile myself to reality: *Acknowledging what is*, a core principle of Family Constellations, severed the bond to my rapist that I had been inadvertently nurturing, and allowed me to leave him behind (mentally and emotionally; he was not in my life), with the full responsibility of his actions. Over time, I have even been able to reconcile with my (formerly) estranged father.

For me, Family Constellations was an epiphany, and it has never ceased to be since that first moment I looked into Charlie's eyes. In the nearly eight years I've been practicing, I've worked with well over 1,000 clients and witnessed countless of them experience epiphanies of their own, as well as sustained and life-changing development, growth, and newfound joy. The vast majority of them came to me after they'd "tried everything else." Struggling with difficult family and romantic relationships, unfulfilling careers, persistent depression and anxiety, the aftereffects of traumas in their own lives, or the sense that *something just isn't right*, they were desperate for their own big shift. And in countless instances, Family Constellations finally flipped that switch for them—not only revealing the unseen family dynamics that stymied them but also empowering them with the tools to disrupt those dynamics for good and write their own singular story going forward.

Some clients I've seen only once, some a handful of times, others work holistically on an array of issues for a year or two, others come for periodic "tune-ups," each according to his or her need. Regardless of the duration of my therapeutic relationship with clients, they e-mail regularly—from within days of a session to months later, then ongoing over the years—to report back happy news of their lives in the wake of the work they've done in Family Constellations: successful career changes, creative breakthroughs, the birth of a child, the cathartic end of a marriage, the bliss of a genuine and healthy love match, a repaired relationship with a parent or sibling. My clients have experienced reconciliation: with loved ones, with the fractured self, with the past, with the possibility of a future over which they have complete agency.

Yet as many people as I do see in my private practice, I wish I could help even more. I'm a passionate ambassador for the power of Family Constellations. I want people from all walks of life (not just those who can access counseling) to benefit from its potent and transformative insights and its ability to dramatically shift our behaviors and beliefs for the better. In-person constellations are of course remarkable, but the fundamental—and life-changing— principles of Family Constellations are accessible, and applicable, beyond the borders of a knowing field.

While my clients' constellations have been tremendous vehicles of change, it has been our work exploring the philosophy and perspective of Family Constellations that has brought them profound and lasting change. Though Family Constellations *therapy* necessarily takes place person-to-person, in one-on-one or group settings, an embrace of Family Constellations' *core principles* has the power to radically shift one's life, without ever experiencing a constellation or setting foot in a facilitator's office. No one can "constellate" themselves—but, through embracing the *philosophy* of Family Constellations, you can empower yourself to recognize the hold on you that your family system possesses; you can learn to disentangle yourself from the destinies of others; you can live intentionally; and you can experience hugely transformative growth, rejecting false narratives about who you are, where you come from, and where you are going, and become free to write your own authentic stories going forward.

That's what I want for you, and that's why I wrote this book. This is not a "how to constellate yourself in seven easy steps" guide (if you do see that book anywhere, *run*) or an exhaustive, comprehensive manual on Family Constellations. Instead, I like to think of it as a "handbook for the soul"—a field guide to the Family Constellations philosophy, its core principles, and their everyday applications—that I hope empowers you with profoundly practical and inspiring tools to take ownership of your life.

In each of the six chapters that follow, together we'll explore a core concept and a core principle of Family Constellations, discovering how to apply the family systems perspective to your own life, so that you can recognize entanglements, disentangle yourself from intergenerational trauma, and work toward healing your own pain—so that you can achieve your own big shift.

You'll encounter a combination of client examples and stories from my own journey, one replete with family secrets and late-life revelations that have challenged some of my long-held beliefs about who I am and where I come from, which Family Constellations has enabled me to navigate with (relative) equanimity. In every chapter, carefully designed affirmations and multiple exercises will help you actively engage with and experience the benefits of Family Constellations in a concrete way for deep healing and lasting change. You can say the affirmations out loud or silently. You can also write them down. Whatever resonates the most with you is the best thing to do. Trust yourself. You can repeat them once a day or several times a day.

In *Connected Fates, Separate Destinies*, you will learn how to:

- Recognize family system patterns and disrupt them
- Heal the inner child, and parent the adult self
- Release limiting beliefs and behaviors

- Dissolve trauma bonds that entangle us with the past
- Reconcile the past and the present, for a whole and integrated self
- Arrive at a place of personal peace within the family system
- Craft future-facing narratives that empower you to live authentically

Our family system impacts the cornerstones of our lives: career, finances, love, and health. The patterns we display in each area link back to the unique dynamics of our family systems. When needs were not met (in our lives or in the lives of those who came before us), on a subconscious level we learned to repeat unhealthy behavior patterns in order to fill the gaps of unmet needs. When we heal the foundation of our being—our family system—we heal every area of our life. Recognizing the pains of our ancestors, acknowledging rejected individuals in our family system, and allowing them to be seen is our ticket to freedom.

Just a few days ago, as I sat in my office late one evening answering e-mails, I got a new message ping. It was one of my clients, Isabelle, letting me know she was opening her own yoga studio. When I met Isabelle several years earlier, she had been working in finance for almost 10 years. Her career wasn't advancing as she had hoped, despite her best efforts, and she was frustrated and increasingly despondent.

Isabelle had been born into a wealthy family—her father was a hedge fund manager and they wanted for nothing. Then at 15, her father's hedge fund collapsed. Not only did the family lose everything, but Isabelle's mother and father divorced in the aftermath, as her father's whole house of cards collapsed: He was sent to jail, and an affair he'd been having came to light—as did the son he had fathered from it. Isabelle acknowledged that the experience had been devastating. She insisted she had no attachment to her father (they were estranged) and that she had gone into finance because she found it genuinely interesting . . . and wanted to make a lot of money. Her career was middling at best, however, and she had been passed over for promotions repeatedly. She also struck me as joyless. I asked Isabelle what she did for fun, what made her happy.

Isabelle paused. Her body language shifted noticeably. She uncrossed her arms, which had been defensively shielding her chest. Her shoulders dropped. "Yoga," she said. She went on to tell me that in addition to her regular practice, she had done a yoga teacher training and had a fantasy of becoming a yoga teacher. "Why is that a fantasy?" I asked her. "I can't make money and support myself being a yoga teacher," she said, her tone indicating that it was worrisome that this wasn't obvious to me.

Before her first constellation, I asked what issue she wanted to work on. She answered, "I want to succeed in my career." Though Isabelle seemed surprised when the constellation laid bare her entanglement with her father, I was not; the loss of the family fortune had precipitated a divorce, which had led to his exclusion in her family system. Isabelle's entanglement with her father sought not only to repair the system but to restore what she had lost. Though the entanglement was not revelatory per se, it showed how Isabelle had taken on her father's fate and its destiny, in conflict with her own. She could not succeed in finance because it was not her destiny. She had misidentified her issue. Over a series of sessions, Isabelle was able to surrender her narratives around success and money and to reintegrate her father into her family system, releasing her anger and fear. Shortly after our last conversation, Isabelle began teaching yoga part-time. Not long after, as her classes drew more and more students, she was able to quit her finance job and teach full-time. Reading her most recent update, I was moved that Isabelle's "fantasy" had become her reality.

Of course, I'd love everyone who reads this to experience an Isabelle-style transformation, and I wish I could work directly with every person drawn to *Connected Fates, Separate Destinies* to make that happen. But I'm content—*excited*—knowing that through the narrative guidance, techniques, and exercises in the book, you will be empowered to examine your family system critically, identify your real issues, and work toward resolving them, for your own major ditching-finance-and-doing-yoga breakthroughs . . . to move from fantasy to reality.

If you're ready to take accountability for your life, then I promise, *Connected Fates, Separate Destinies* is for you. You don't need to have any special access to family history or genealogy; its effectiveness is not contingent upon unearthing family secrets. You can learn to affirm your ancestors and release unconscious loyalties and misplaced responsibilities, even if you cannot explicitly name them. Simply through recognizing the struggles of our ancestors, we acknowledge that our pains are a collective wound that never healed. When we acknowledge our family members for the traumas they experienced, accept them as they are, and give them a place to belong, we experience a deep personal healing.

All you need to get the most out of this book is a desire to be happy and a willingness to do the work to get there. Bert Hellinger called happiness "an achievement of the soul." By this he meant that true happiness is the experience of fulfillment, which can be attained only through the work of authentic self-expression— work that is active, that has strength and energy. "We live in our works," he said, "and that happiness is different from the happiness of a party."

The power of Family Constellations, the happiness it has to offer—as we'll experience together—is the ways in which it teaches us to truly recognize that we are part of a family system and that events in the system, which predate us, may have caused us to act in a way that was beyond our conscious control. But going forward, liberated from the narratives of inherited traumas and disordered family system dynamics, we get to tell our own authentic story. We get to experience an achievement of the soul.

CHAPTER 1

Origin Stories

The Family System

E ach of us has a family. Every family exists in its own unique ecosystem: an intersection of history, culture, beliefs, and genetics. Every family has a heritage it passes down from generation to generation. We might share the same last name and sometimes even the first name as our family members or ancestors, as well as the same DNA, roots, culture, and stories. An invisible yarn links us together through time, a sort of internal family memory, so that the force of past events may tug on us in the here and now, even if we ourselves never directly experienced the things that were impactful for those who came before us.

And regardless of its shape—motherless, fatherless, only child, adopted, blended, "conventional" or not—or our relationship to it, we each also have a story we tell ourselves about that family. We know its characters and its plot by heart; we know who the villains are, who is right and who is wrong. At the center of the story is the self: where we've come from, where we are going, what we deserve.

For some, the story might sound like, "I can't get close to anyone because my mother never showed me love," or "My parents always struggled financially, and now my guilt at outshining them prevents me from succeeding professionally." My story was of a once united family splintered first by divorce and then further fragmented by my father's abandonment—and my subsequent struggle to feel at home in the world, my heart and trust broken, alienated from love and security. *My father left me; I must not be worthy of love.*

These stories are often unconscious and thus their implications obscured to us. We become stuck in the narrative and repeat it over and over. When I first came to Family Constellations, I had already been in therapy for years. Like a lot of my own clients now, I wasn't consciously aware of the narrative I had crafted because I treated that narrative not as a story of my own making but as a set of facts about my life, turning over their different facets, seeking to reveal how I had been shaped by them, so I could understand what was "wrong with me"—and who to blame. I thought knowing this would help me "fix" myself, help me avoid the mistakes I'd been making in my life and relationships. But, despite how fiercely I sought insight, liberation, and relief . . . they failed to arrive in any meaningful way.

Instead, my story, in which my father leaving illustrated my unworthiness as an object of male love, compelled me to create a supporting story, equally flawed. I tried to soothe the wound with the balm of my "independence." After all, I came from a line of incredibly strong women; I did not need to trust or rely on men. My romantic life suffered profoundly as a result, and I made a lot of poor choices.

Sound familiar? Even after years of therapy, so many of us find ourselves still stuck in, or making slow progress away from, the same old limiting beliefs and behaviors. Don't get me wrong—I would never deny the value of traditional talk therapy, whether it's psychodynamic, cognitive behavioral, or another approach. For many of us, therapy is the first environment in which we've ever been free to discuss our feelings openly, and doing so can help us explore and identify *how* they impact our thoughts and moods. Therapists occupy a unique space that family and friends can't (and shouldn't) fill: They are impartial listeners who are still on our side ("our side" being the side of achieving better mental health) and highly trained to deal with distorted perception. Therapy might be the first time our experience is affirmed, and thus validated. And, of course, when our experience is affirmed and validated, we feel seen, which is crucial to healing.

The thing is, traditional talk therapy is often premised on reaffirming our existing narratives about our family, treating those stories as a source for better understanding ourselves. *But what if our stories are the problem, and the premise itself is flawed? What if we've gotten them all wrong? What if we're not even reading the right book?*

Humans are born storytellers. Narrative is our magic. It imposes order on chaos, infuses the arbitrary with meaning, and makes time travelers of us all. But our family stories are not an impartial record of what happened to us; they are a narrative of how we *feel* about what happened to us, our *thoughts* about the players and the events, further colored by inherited attitudes and beliefs. They are unreliable narratives, oriented around the individual, anchored in a subjective viewpoint.

Family Constellations decisively rejects this mode of storytelling. It interrupts our narrative habits: our reliance on casting people in our lives as villains and heroes, and our insistence on seeing our lives as a linearly unfolding plot determined by cause and effect. Family Constellations challenges us to face our past from a place of suspended moral judgment. In other words, it demands that we set aside a need to determine who or what was right or wrong, which requires interpretation. Instead, we focus only on *what* happened, not on why or what it means. We seek to understand and abide by the impartial forces that govern human kinship relationships, that order and rule what Family Constellations calls the **"family system."**

Let's pause here for a minute and reflect on what a system *is*, anyway. To get really basic, let's say that a system comprises a group of individual components that form a unified whole, greater than the sum of its parts. Those individual components are dependent on each other to function, and the system is powered by the dynamics of that *interdependence*. A system is all about the integrity of its structure, about the *interconnectedness* of its components. Systems are about the collective, versus the individual.

In the Family Constellations model, every individual is born not just into a family but into a family *system*, a sort of energetic network or structure comprised of every member of that family, living or dead, going back over the generations (and extending into the future). Family members are interconnected across generations in this system by the family soul, by what Bert Hellinger called "the movement of love"—the life force with which each generation imbues the next. In a healthy family system, that flow of love, of life force energy, is unencumbered and courses forward in time from one generation to the next. The dynamics of the family, rather than the isolated actions of one individual, determine the health of the system.

All systems seek balance. In a family system, equilibrium depends primarily on two principles: **order and belonging**. First, every member of the family system has his or her rightful position—or *order*—in that network, the place where they fit and interact most naturally, that upholds the structure of the system. Though we each have our own unique order in our family systems (in other words, no one else can take our place), the overall order of family members is, in a sense, the same in every family: a matter of precedence—who came first. In a constellation, a facilitator will always initially arrange the participants so that the representative for the client's father stands behind him on his right, while the representative for the mother stands behind the client on his left. Both of them are followed by their own parents, grandparents, and ancestors behind them in the same pattern. I love this image because it illustrates the potential strength the family system affords us, the support at our backs that allows us to face forward with confidence. Whenever you feel overwhelmed, have a seat, close your eyes, take a few deep breaths, and call on those prior generations. Lean on them. Trust them. Sense the inherent bend toward order in the family system. When systems are in order, we feel relief, peace, a sense of things working smoothly together.

Part of orderliness is *belonging*. As I said, every member of a family has a unique place in it (their order in the system) that no one else can fill, and thus the right to belong to that family. The desire to belong is one of our most fundamental of human urges. Children will do almost anything to ensure that they belong to their parents; they experience a kind of "crazy" or blind love and loyalty, regardless of the parents in question. (Often, we unwittingly carry that loyalty—however misguided—into adulthood.) The drive to belong is part of what binds us to our family system and to each other; it helps keep the system intact. Part of belonging is each member's right to their own fate (the cards they're dealt) and its destiny (how they play those cards), i.e., their ownership of and responsibility for their actions and their consequences.

These rights aren't a matter of morals or ethics. They are more akin to natural law. When disorder occurs (when precedence isn't honored or a child takes the place of a parent, for example), or a family member experiences severe trauma or is excluded from and denied belonging in the family system (usually as a result of a traumatic event), or their fate isn't respected (allowed to rest with them), the system—the network—can no longer function properly.

A system will always try to make itself complete again, functional, in balance. In an effort to repair the damage—to restore the integrity of the network—the family system will seek to employ members of new generations to take the place of or mitigate the harm of past generations, members who will take up traumatized, missing, or excluded family members' fates and "correct" what cannot, of course, be corrected. As my teacher Suzi Tucker once said, every child is "a next best chance" to restore a family system's integrity. This dynamic is called an *entanglement*, and entanglements—inherited traumas that drive us to repeat the patterns of the past—are at the root of so much of our pain. We reenact dysfunctional dynamics, blindly loyal soldiers recruited by a system desperately trying to right itself. That's why one of the key takeaways of Family Constellations to keep close at heart is the simple mantra: *It did not start with me.*

What's fascinating is that new research being done in epigenetics is increasingly supporting this systemic view, in which our individual struggles are a by-product of a deeper shared family legacy, by demonstrating the inheritability of trauma at the cellular level. Epigenetics is the study of the mechanisms that switch genes "on" and "off"—in other words, the *environmental* and *experiential* factors that control gene expression, or which genes are active or inactive. Certain types of trauma, such as starvation, may "shut off" the expression of certain genes without changing the underlying DNA, and those "instructions" can be passed down from parent to child without any alteration to the gene itself. We know we inherit our brown eyes biologically and that our families may also "pass on" their attitudes, customs, and beliefs, but our bodies themselves may carry the legacies of what our ancestors endured.

More than 70 years after enduring famine in utero, the cohort of children born during the Dutch Hunger Winter provided startlingly clear evidence of epigenetics at work. In September 1944, the Nazis began blocking food supplies to the occupied Netherlands as punishment for assisting a failed Allied campaign. By the time the Netherlands was liberated in May 1945, more than 20,000 Dutch citizens had died of starvation. Dutch women who gave birth early during the famine had babies who were born underweight, but who eventually caught up to normal weight. On the other hand, babies born to women who became pregnant later in the famine and gave birth after the war were born normal weight. They *seemed* to have escaped the detrimental effects of malnutrition in utero (this made sense, given that babies gain most of their weight in the third trimester of pregnancy). In the long term, though, this group suffered increased rates of obesity, elevated cholesterol levels, and other metabolic problems in middle age. Scientists who collected blood samples from this cohort and from their siblings born before and long after the war discovered something fascinating: Unlike their siblings, people who were in utero during the Hunger Winter shared the same "silenced" gene, PIM3, which is involved in how the body burns fuel. Though a fetus often more than triples its weight during the third trimester of pregnancy, it is during the first trimester that the majority of fetal development occurs, when "cell programming" takes place. For these children, their mother's experience of starvation (an environmental factor) became written on their very cells.

In Family Constellations, the first goal is to make the invisible visible. Once you are able to see the dynamics in your family system and identify entanglements, you are empowered to disrupt them, liberating not only yourself but also members of subsequent generations from their hold. The second goal is resolution: By recognizing every member of the system (granting them belonging) and allowing them their rightful place (restoring order), you release any unconscious loyalties you may have been carrying. This way, you no longer shoulder responsibilities that are not your own—or the behaviors, thoughts, and emotions that doing so can produce.

Systems thinking asks us to recognize that we are part of something bigger than ourselves, that our problems are not ours alone, and that we are interconnected with others in a web of reverberating patterns and dynamics. Becoming a "systems thinker" isn't easy, but it is a radical gift you can give yourself. Most of us are addicted to a need to be right when it comes to our hurt and pain. We're committed to seeing other people as characters in a story in which we star. But holding on to that story can mean holding on to negative thoughts, behaviors, or events we use to justify our current choices, behaviors, and relationships, hampering us from taking responsibility for our lives. When you become a systems thinker, you decenter the self in favor of a networked way of seeing, necessarily shifting focus from the individual to the collective. This helps us build empathy not only for others but also for ourselves, which, in turn, helps us reframe our origin stories—those narratives about where we come from and where we're going, that are inevitably about what we deserve or don't deserve, our worth or lovability.

In my case, when I began examining my family system apart from the cloud of my judgments around individuals' actions within it, I saw a clear pattern of abandonment emerge across generations. Instead of clinging to *"My father left me; I must not be worthy of love,"* I was eventually able to stop rejecting and judging my father (excluding him from my family system) and resolve the entanglement. This didn't mean I approved of his actions or absolved him of responsibility, but it did mean I accepted the reality of what he had done without an overlay of what it "meant"; I was able to understand it as a dynamic of the family system, rather than as a reflection of my value as a person. In doing so, I put the past to rest. When you've put the past to rest, you no longer have to turn your back on the present, and you can face the future on your terms, no longer caught up in narratives about harm done and what that says about you.

It gets tricky here, I admit. It almost seems like an impossible contradiction: In order to move beyond the family, and beyond your stories about your family, you must accept your family. Not embrace or even like them, but accept that they do, indeed, belong to the system. This is an act of love because it helps restore the integrity of the system. Bringing the system into balance allows the movement of love, of life force energy, to follow its natural and intended course: forward.

We separate from the past but not from people. Truly stepping out of our family of origin comes not through rejection but through acceptance, not through an obsessive rehashing of the past but through an active choosing of the present. We reconcile what *is* with what *was* so we can access what *can be*—leaving behind the heavy weight of our old stories and allowing us to write new ones, to fully be the authors of our own lives on the path of our highest destiny.

MEDITATION: Everyone Has a Place

This meditation is meant to help build a visceral sense of the family system's ideal order and belonging. Throughout, I refer to family members who may or may not be part of your life, people you may or may not have known. All of our families are unique. When your experience differs from my words, I invite you to visualize the *archetype* instead, e.g., the archetype of the grandmother as wise woman, as storyteller, as matriarch. This is especially critical in relation to our biological parents. Many of us have parents who are not our biological parents: We may be adopted; we may have caregivers who stepped up and in for an absent parent; our parent or parents may have used a sperm or egg donor, etc. In these cases, we must still include our biological parents, as they are the source of our life. [Note: I suggest you read the meditation through first, and if you're comfortable doing so, use your smartphone or other device to record yourself reading it. That way, you can listen to the meditation and focus on your visualizations without having to interrupt yourself to check the page for what comes next. If you would like, you may also listen to this meditation in the audiobook format of this title.]

Find a comfortable spot, a space where you can feel peaceful and at ease. You may sit cross-legged or, if you are seated on a sofa or chair, ground your feet on the floor. Allow your palms to rest facing up on your thighs—this is a posture of openness and receptivity.

Take a few deep breaths and close your eyes. Visualize your mother and invite her to stand behind your left shoulder. Feel her presence. Next, visualize your father and invite him to join you behind your right shoulder. Feel his presence. This is where they belong: behind you, supporting you, guiding you. You can adjust the distance between you and them. It is important that you feel comfortable too. However, they have to stay behind you.

Now, visualize your maternal grandparents. Invite them to take their places behind your mother. Visualize your paternal grandparents. Invite them to take their places behind your father. Again, this is where they belong: behind your mom and behind your dad, supporting them, guiding them, and loving them for who they are.

Visualize your great-grandparents and invite them to take their places behind your grandparents. Stretching out behind them are your ancestors. Your entire family is there, extending back through time, an endless and unbroken chain. Through them flows your legacy, your cultural and genetic inheritances. Everyone and everything they encompass is right behind you. This is your heritage. This is your story. And everyone belongs; everyone is seen; everyone is heard. Everyone is recognized. Everyone has a place. Everyone is important, as you are important, as you have a place too.

See if you can connect to your inner child, the little boy or little girl who you used to be. Where is she? What is he doing? How old is she? Does he look sad, lonely, happy? Ask them silently, *What can I do for you? How can I help you?* Take one of their hands and come back to your place in front of your parents. And tell them, silently, *My little girl, my little boy, this is your place. This is where you belong. You are not here to take care of Mom or Dad; you are here to take care of yourself. And for now, I will be the one taking care of you. You can lean on me. You can trust me. I'm not going anywhere without you anymore.*

If you have older siblings, please ask them to join you on your right side—as your siblings are of roughly the same generation, they will stand next to you, not behind you. If you have younger siblings, please ask them to join you on your left side. Include any half siblings. If you are aware of any pregnancies your mother had that were miscarried or aborted, please also invite them to join you.

If you have a stepparent and he or she is important to you and part of your life, invite them to join you. Your stepfather should stand next to your mother and your stepmother next to your father. Similarly, if you have stepsiblings with whom you are close, you may invite them to stand alongside your other siblings.

Now take a few steps forward, holding the hand of your inner child, looking unhesitatingly forward. Your destiny is in front of you. Step toward it, embrace it, welcome it, knowing that your family is right behind you, supporting and guiding you.

If you are in a committed relationship, visualize your partner and invite them to join you. If you're a heterosexual woman, your man will stand to your right; if you're a heterosexual man, your woman will stand to your left. If you are in a same-sex or nonbinary couple, you can choose to place your partner either on your right or left side, whichever feels best.

Finally, if you have children, please invite them to stand in front of you (including any miscarried or aborted pregnancies—again, because everyone belongs). You are in charge of this next generation, protecting and guiding them and doing your best to love them as they are. (If you share children with an ex-partner, invite your ex to join you on the left side of your current partner, if you have one. Otherwise, follow the earlier guidelines. Your marriage might have ended, but as co-parents, you will forever be a family.)

Feel the strength coming from your past and the profound attachment to your present life, deeply grounded and loved. You belong, you have a place, and everyone in your family has a place too. That's the beauty of the family system. You can always lean on your ancestors to recharge your battery. Take a few more minutes to feel that deep connection with your heritage. You are whole and complete, and that's the gift that you will pass on to the next generation. With every new generation, there is another chance to do better, to love more, to respect more, and to accept more.

When you feel ready, very slowly and gently open your eyes.

EXERCISE:

"I Am Because We Are"—Becoming a Systems Thinker

Ubuntu, often translated as "I am because we are," is both a belief and a values system, a set of practices and a way of being in the world that emphasizes our interconnectedness and honors it. Archbishop Desmond Tutu described *ubuntu* this way: "A person with *ubuntu* is open and available to others, affirming of others, does not feel threatened that others are able and good, for he or she has a proper self-assurance that comes from knowing that he or she belongs in a greater whole and is diminished when others are humiliated or diminished, when others are tortured or oppressed." Bert Hellinger first encountered the pan-African philosophy working with Zulu peoples in South Africa, and it came to deeply inform his work: In Family Constellations, we are constantly challenged to see ourselves as part of a greater whole, as a collective of interconnected transgenerational family members. This way of seeing is what I've called variously "systems thinking," "the systemic view," and "a networked way of seeing."

The thing is, this way of thinking can be extremely difficult to embrace—let alone practice—after a lifetime of training that, especially in the United States, emphasizes and celebrates rugged individualism. I think it is important to acknowledge that habits, including habitual ways of thinking, take time to undo. Learning a new way of thinking isn't something that happens overnight; building the muscle of systems thinking takes commitment, time, and practice. One of the best ways to build that muscle is to practice what I like to think of as "everyday interconnectedness." This means getting outside yourself and starting where you are, both by focusing on opportunities for prosocial behavior in day-to-day life and looking for the ways in which we already experience interconnectedness. When we train ourselves to start seeing and practicing interconnectedness all around us, it becomes much more natural to accept our family as an interconnected system.

What follows are ideas for getting you into a daily practice of interconnectedness, grounded in empathy, gratitude, and kindness. You can mix and match these however feels right to you. The point isn't to create a list of tasks for yourself—interconnectedness shouldn't feel onerous; the point is for it to feel natural, because it is. The plan here is to simply bring you into awareness of that interconnectedness, so that eventually it is second nature to operate from that vantage point.

GET OUTSIDE, NO DISTRACTIONS: The greatest system we are all a part of is nature, especially as it intersects with humanity. If it is safe for you to do so, I strongly suggest that you take a walk every day, without headphones, whatever the weather. Ideally, the sole purpose of the walk is just to walk, for about 30 minutes or so (if you have longer, great). If you live somewhere with easy access to natural beauty, great. But that's not necessary. Nature exists all around us. And not every day is beautiful, anyway.

While you walk, pay attention to your body and its relationship to the world around you. Feel the air on your face, your skin. Is it cool, hot, wet, dry? Listen to the ambient noise. What do you hear? What do you smell? Exhaust? Damp earth? Hot concrete? Salt water? What do you see? Really look at what you're passing— all of it, ugly and beautiful—especially where nature and the man-made come together, such as weeds coming up through the sidewalk, neighborhood gardens, etc.

It's actually lovely to take a walk like this with another person, but only if you can agree to do so in silence. When you're done, you can talk about what you both experienced. The enforced silence is also a beautiful experiment in intimacy and awareness of the other. It disrupts our habit of filling silences, and part of what we become truly aware of is the other person's presence—the sound of their breath, their footfalls, the fabric of a jacket swishing.

CONNECT WITH SPIRITUALITY: You don't have to be remotely religious to be spiritual, at least the way I define it. You can identify as atheist or agnostic or nothing at all. By spirituality, I mean that sense of being part of something bigger than yourself, of experiencing awe, or of coming in contact with the spark of creation. And yes, this is possible in everyday life, though maybe not every day. When we connect with spirituality, we experience transcendence. If you are religious, you may of course experience this in temple, church, synagogue, or mosque. You can also experience awe by getting outside (sunset often does the trick), as above. But in a daily way, awe often comes when we experience the transcendence of the human spirit through art. When we experience art, be it a piece of music, a passage of writing, a painting or sculpture, etc., we experience the magic of connecting with another soul across space and time.

Make time every day to listen to a song you find moving (while doing nothing else) or to read a chapter in a novel. Set aside time to do this; plan for it. Genuinely make it a part of your schedule. Before or after, really think about the person/people on the other side of the creation. You might not experience straight-up awe every day, sure. But you are remembering that nothing exists in isolation. And though they may not be daily activities, live shows, concerts, museum exhibits, and theater performances are also incredible opportunities to experience interconnectedness, with the artists, the audience, and the human spirit that animates it all.

JUST DO SOMETHING: Volunteerism is great, of course, but there are a lot of bars to begin volunteering and it can be time-consuming. Bystander training is a fantastic resource to help you learn how to directly or indirectly safely de-escalate, intervene, or change course when you witness harassment in daily life. Rather than feeling frozen in place, you can, through bystander training, feel empowered and capable of standing up for someone else, of putting interconnectedness into action. But you can also engage in small daily acts of decency, asking yourself, *How can I help make this experience better for everyone?* Can you offer your seat on public transportation? Let another vehicle merge in front of you? Be patient in a slow line? Be polite with service people and customer support representatives, regardless of extenuating circumstances?

Ask yourself, *What will dumping on this person (who probably has little to no power themselves) actually accomplish besides making them feel bad?* Remember and believe that everything you do, or don't do, has an impact on others.

REMEMBER, IT'S NOT ABOUT YOU: You don't have to take someone else's shit, but remember that it's almost never about you (unless you are being an asshole). This might seem anathema to interconnectedness, but it's really not. It's about setting aside your ego and remembering that there are other forces at play that can affect how someone perceives a situation or how they treat you. Again, this doesn't mean you should accept abusive or toxic behaviors from others. But it does mean that with regular-old low-level rudeness, irritation, etc., you don't have to engage or meet the person where they are. Take a breath and center yourself. You can walk away, end the conversation, draw on your compassion, extend empathy. You can choose to see the other person as a human susceptible to mood or caught up in their own patterns, rather than take their actions as a personal offense. This is *especially* helpful with family members, with whom we tend to react automatically.

Acknowledging What Is

Would you rather be right or be happy? That's probably the first question I should have told you to ask yourself before even starting this book. Because your answer must be "happy." And the harsh reality is, the two are often incompatible. Shifting to thinking from a systemic viewpoint gets us at least halfway to happy, for sure. But you don't become a systemic thinker overnight, no matter how much you try to will it. The ability to be a systemic thinker—to grasp the nature of the family system from that place of suspended moral judgment—starts with a commitment to, and a practice of, *acknowledging what is.*

What does that mean? Reality is never wrong, even when it sucks. As a facilitator or constellation participant, the first thing you learn in Family Constellations is the importance of acknowledging, respecting, and accepting your family **as it is**. In other words, you must agree to reality; you must be able to acknowledge who your family members are, what happened, and to whom, *apart from any meaning or intention you ascribe to those events or people.* That's what allows us to apprehend the dynamics in a system; that's what allowed me to admit my father back into my family system. We are able to do so when we stand in that place of "suspended moral judgment," the neutral space that is separate from our individual belief systems, where we leave behind right and wrong. In this space, we strip ourselves of our stories (our perceptions of what happened) and are free to look with love—in other words, with the energy of life force—at the bare facts, at what really happened.

When we'd rather be right than give up judgment, we create a block to resolution, because judgment blinds us to being able to see the dynamics in a system. Judgment is predicated on interpretation, on the conscious mind's need to be in control. Needing to be in control is refusing to grow. There is a childishness to it: Children, who have very little control over their lives, grasp tightly to whatever they can control; they tend to resist change and do badly with transitions. The problem is that 90 percent of the time we are grown-ups still thinking with a child's mindset. As adults, healing happens when we change our perception from a childlike mentality to understanding the broader story before our lifetime. This approach encourages us to accept and respect our past, instead of disowning or romanticizing it, both of which are aspects of control. And control is always a form of resistance. Awakening happens when we change our perception, accept what is, and surrender—or consent—to reality.

So, *acknowledging what is* is a process of *accepting* and *consenting* to reality. When we accept what is, we step away from our narratives and our need to be right. Instead, we simply agree to the reality of what happened, without judgment. Let me be clear: This does not mean we are agreeing that what happened should have happened, only that it did. When we agree with reality, we can then consent to it *and stop arguing with it*—stop attempting to control it. We are not consenting to our feelings about what happened to us; we are consenting to the fact that the past cannot be unwritten.

When we consent to what is, we finally cede control in an arena in which we have never had any actual control. Too often we go to therapy seeking confirmation, to feel *right* in our suffering. We want validation that our mother was wrong, that our boss is the problem, and that holding onto anger serves us. But we will never find real healing in the need to be right, which is rooted in fear, self-protection, and the impulse to preserve our deep-rooted stories, which we believe are our identities. The need to be right is a need to be in control, and it centers us in every story, making it difficult if not impossible to see the bigger picture of the family system.

When we acknowledge what is, when we agree with and consent to reality without judgment, we experience a clarity of perception that is liberating. We are able to perceive that we are part of a family system and can focus on understanding its *dynamics*, rather than on the actions of individuals alone. In doing so, we acknowledge our ancestors' place in that system and affirm their right to belong, honoring their fate and leaving their responsibilities at their feet, where they belong, unraveling the binding threads of entanglement.

Acknowledging what is is an incredible tool for life. When we acknowledge what is, we take into account all that has happened. In doing so, we are forced to pause. We have to forgo our old habits of thought, our ego-based reactions. We get as close to an objective perspective as is possible for subjective beings like ourselves. Objectivity allows us to step outside ourselves, to better comprehend others not just as equals but as equally *real*. When our perception of the world is centered in and filtered through the self (subjectivity), others are reduced to supporting players in the movie of our life, in which we are the star. When our perception of the world is centered outside the self (objectivity), as much as that is possible, we understand that others are the stars of their own movies. Objectivity helps us step out of ourselves and into the other. Acknowledging what is fosters our empathy. It is not that it insists that there is no right or wrong, but it reminds us that we are not always the best arbiters of that distinction—that other people possess different perspectives that they embrace as "right" with just as much fervor, and that in many cases neither may be provable.

Within our families, this impartial view widens our field of vision—we can more clearly perceive not only the events of our own lives but also those of our ancestors, and the effects of those events. When we can bear witness to our ancestors and honor their fate, we are better able to bear witness to the flow of life, to the movement of love. This also means we are better able to bear witnesses to experiences of *all* kinds, without assuming victimhood, assigning blame, or making judgments. It opens us to a greater spectrum of human experience, and empowers us to come from a place of love—that is, a place where we accept people as they are, without wanting anything from them. We are able to recognize and honor their humanity, regardless of their actions, the responsibility for which we leave with them. When we are able to do this for our own ancestors, we can finally draw on the strength and accept with grace the goodness and resources they do have to offer us, no matter how difficult the legacy.

AFFIRMATIONS

I belong to my family system.

When I acknowledge what was, I can be at peace with what is.

I consent to what is, I cede control, I embrace my own fate.

EXERCISE: Overcoming Resistance

Practicing acceptance in our daily lives can help us with over-coming resistance to the reality of more difficult events when they occur. Acceptance is a tricky beast—many of us resist it because of what we think acceptance means: weakness, surrender, quitting, passivity. So let's tackle those head-on. Acceptance is not weakness; it takes great strength to confront an uncomfortable or painful reality. Acceptance is not surrendering or quitting; it is choosing to stop pouring your energy into a void. Acceptance is not passivity; it is an active assertion of your real agency. Remember, refusing to accept reality doesn't change it. Acceptance is not about toxic positivity, and it's definitely not "everything happens for a reason." It's the opposite. It's acknowledging that bad things happen and there doesn't need to be a reason or a positive out-come. Pain is a part of life, but we don't need to add suffering to that pain fighting against it. Here are some strategies to practice acceptance every day:

STOP STRUGGLING AGAINST NEGATIVE EMOTIONS: *Struggle* is the key word here. Resistance is a struggle. Practice sitting with a bad feeling—shame, anger, fear, guilt, embarrassment—rather than avoiding or attempting to neutralize it. Did you make a mistake at work? What happens when you just let yourself feel that embarrass-ment? Guess what? You're still there on the other side of that feel-ing. The feeling isn't you; you aren't the feeling. It's a response to a moment in time, not a life sentence. Don't pile suffering onto pain by fighting it.

NOTICE YOUR THOUGHTS: You're stuck in traffic and late to an important appointment. Take a breath and listen to yourself. What is run-ning through your head? Catastrophizing? A litany of pejoratives about the drivers around you? Berating yourself? Actively shift your thoughts to a mantra such as, "This situation is upsetting and frustrating. There is nothing I can do about it right now. I don't like it, but it is what it is." Acceptance isn't about approval. You don't have to like reality, only to acknowledge it.

DETACH YOURSELF FROM OUTCOMES: Set goals and do your best to achieve them, but once you have done so remind yourself that you cannot control everything. Let go of the connection between your self-worth and your success or failure prior to the outcome. Remind yourself that no matter how it turns out, your happiness is not dependent on the outcome.

SHIFT FOCUS FROM WHAT YOU CAN'T CONTROL TO WHAT YOU CAN: Like I said, acceptance is not about quitting. You can't change the past (and so often, like when you're stuck in traffic, you can't change the present)—but you can change how you feel about it, you can change your circumstances, and you can change the future. Let go of should haves and would haves. You can't change that a partner was unfaithful (and you can't change or control another person). But rather than ruminating on it or holding on to resentment or perpetually using the infidelity to emotionally bully a partner, you can choose to end the relationship, you can choose to try counseling, or you can try to rebuild trust in good faith.

Honoring Our Ancestors

In Family Constellations, we talk a lot about the diverse dynamics and entanglements between the past and the present and how so much of healing depends on acknowledging and accepting the past—and finding the right distance from it. With individuals in our family system, this means acknowledging and *respecting* their fate. Respecting a family member's fate does not mean admiring it. It means having due regard for it—giving it appropriate consideration. When we respect the fate of our ancestors, we have due regard for the fact that their fate is not our fate;

we do not interfere in it; we recognize those boundaries. The word *respect* itself stems from the Latin *respectus*, which means "to look back." It quite literally implies distance between the subject and the object of that regard. We respect that their fate is what it is and that it belongs to them. When we understand that their fate belongs to them, we also understand that it is their responsibility. We leave it at their feet and we do not take up their destiny; we don't try to suppress or "rewrite" what was.

Respecting the fates of our ancestors can be extremely difficult, however, when their legacies—and thus our own—are complicated by the larger forces of history (which is the case for pretty much every human on Earth). Just as we belong to our family system, our family system belongs to larger systems in turn: community, culture, country, and the countries of our ancestors. These systems are shaped, informed, and animated by forces such as war, violence, conflict, colonization, emigration, immigration, and racial and religious persecution, among others, that can mean our ancestors had extremely difficult fates, sometimes as perpetrators and sometimes as victims in large-scale events.

Whether our ancestors were perpetrators or victims (or as is so often the case, a mix of both), we are often compelled to resist the reality of those pasts. Anyone else remember when a certain A-list actor persuaded the Harvard professor host of a PBS television show to edit out the fact that he had slave owners in the family tree? After leaked e-mails revealed the incident, the megastar explained that he was "embarrassed." On the other end of that spectrum, I have worked with clients whose parents or grandparents survived genocide and never spoke of their experiences—and it was understood by their children to be a verboten topic. The problem is, when we resist or suppress the full picture of our heritage, we resist how we came to be, and thus who we are in all our complexity. It is critical to remember that as much as we may wish things were different, where our ancestors are from, what they did, and what happened to them are unchangeable facts of life. When we resist those facts, we are refusing to acknowledge what is. When we reject the reality of who our ancestors were and what shaped them, we reject life itself.

When we can't account for reality in all its complexity, we also lose the ability to grow and change, to disrupt damaging patterns, and to positively shift the course of the future. Just imagine if that A-list actor had embraced the reality that his ancestor had owned slaves? He could have engaged in a powerful conversation about the need for white Americans to come to real terms with the legacy of slavery in the United States, addressing an audience (his fans) who might otherwise be resistant to such a conversation. The irony is, if he had been open and unashamed from the beginning, he would have been judged far less harshly by the public when the news broke of his successful bid to censor the television episode. It's natural to be ashamed or embarrassed about the immoral and unethical acts of the people in our lineage, of course. We're all only human. But here's what I'd like to remind you of: Fate is always neutral in the sense that we have no control over when, where, or to whom we are born. It is what is. One's fate is not—or need not be—a character judgment. What you *do* with that fate, what destiny you pursue, that's where character emerges.

Even if an individual family member or ancestor was not directly impacted by the larger forces of history, our family systems (and thus ourselves) are still shaped inescapably by those currents of fate. We cannot separate ourselves from them; we belong to our cultures, however uncomfortable that truth may be. The history and culture of the country that is our home is not mutable (neither is that of our ancestors, if we now live elsewhere, as so many of us do). It is what it is. When we do not or cannot acknowledge the fullness of that history, we risk entanglement with its dysfunctional dynamics; we risk perpetuating those dynamics with others and with ourselves. For example, if we benefit from institutionalized racism but refuse to acknowledge that fact or are defensive about it, we only deepen its hold on us and on our culture. Look, I'll say it again: Fate is not a character judgment on *you*. It's just a set of facts. No one is an inherently bad (or good) person just because they are born into a certain system. It becomes a matter of character when you refuse opportunities to understand the system, to acknowledge what is, and to then take action to disrupt negative patterns and create positive change. When we do not or cannot acknowledge the messiness of history, we also miss out on exploiting (in the good way) the resources our cultures *do* have to offer us.

When we do not respect the fate of another, or the currents of fate that power forces such as war, we may end up taking on the fate as if it were our own. If a family member was a victim, we may become a perpetrator in turn to "avenge" the wounds of the past, or we may abdicate authority over our own lives; if we are descended from a perpetrator of violence we may, in our need to repress our guilt or shame, refuse to acknowledge current manifestations of the same, or we may become victims ourselves as an act of "repentance."

Just as *acknowledging what is* is the first step in being able to see your family system with clarity, you must acknowledge what is in your cultural legacy. The super hard part here is how you're supposed to do that from a place of suspended moral judgment, when that legacy may include devastating acts of violence and subjugation, such as colonization, slavery, or genocide. Why would you even want to? Some things are just undeniably evil, bad, immoral, unethical, *fucked up*. Let's get into it. Look, when I write that you need to suspend moral judgment, I do not mean that you must deny morality. Right and wrong are real. *But*, and it's a big but, in order to account for all that has happened in your cultural legacy—and I do mean all, even the ugliest bits— you need to set right and wrong aside *temporarily*. Big emphasis on temporarily, okay? Why do you need to set them aside? Because those categories naturally create inclusion (right) and exclusion (wrong), belonging (right) and rejection (wrong). See where this is going? It isn't possible to take everything into account when your brain is already rejecting certain things as "wrong." We must set these categories aside *temporarily* in order to fully account for what happened, so that we can allow for and *respect* the fate of each ancestor or member of our nation, no matter how hard it might be to stomach that fate. It is only when we respect the fate of our ancestors that we can truly take up our own destinies, both at the individual and cultural levels.

We cannot rectify the past; we can only acknowledge it and then attempt to break its patterns, beginning with ourselves. On the large scale, if we can't do this, we perpetuate the systemic beliefs that uphold exclusionary and oppressive practices such as racism, xenophobia, and classism. On the individual scale, we get stuck in limiting stories about who we are and what we are capable of. When we respect the fate of our ancestors, we change our perspective of our origin stories.

For example, several of my Black and Jewish clients already demonstrate such a relationship to the fates of their ancestors and their complex, multifaceted cultural inheritances. Rather than resist the brutal history of slavery or of the Holocaust, they consent to its reality and include the perpetrators of these atrocities in their systemic view. *Record scratch.* Yikes—did I just write that they include perpetrators in their systemic view?! I understand if you're feeling an instant and intense resistance to that sentence, to the very idea of doing so. Why should anyone want to include agents of genocide in their systemic view? First, it isn't about "wanting"— my clients don't *want* to include those who have harmed them. Instead, it's that they grasp the *interconnectedness* of the fates of victims and perpetrators, the ways in which the lives of their ancestors intersected with those who harmed them and were forever changed as a result. My clients recognize that they cannot argue with reality and that there exists a chain of interlinked events and people that leads to them and to the rich legacy that is their birthright. They do not see their ancestors primarily as victims; they see them as survivors, as people whose beautiful human qualities of resourcefulness, creativity, intelligence, faith, etc., helped them defy a destiny that others tried to impose on them. In turn, they don't see the perpetrators as faceless agents of evil. Rather, they understand them as fallible humans from whom, in representing the worst of us, they can learn deep though discomfiting truths about what leads people to commit evil.

From their families and their cultures, these clients receive "early training" in honoring the fates of previous generations and drawing strength from them, from an origin story that describes perseverance against all odds in the form of persistence, resilience, and survival. Such an origin story powers these clients with the necessary energy and conviction to advocate for change, to work as activists, to fight for a present and future that is radically inclusive. With clients who come from families or groups that perpetrated crimes against others, when they are finally able to reckon with this reality without judgment (such as shame or denial)— when they stop resisting it; when they acknowledge what was and can therefore include these ancestors and this history in their family system—they are lightened rather than burdened. This lightness then actually frees them to do the work to fight for a present and future that is radically inclusive, because they are no longer afraid of what they will see when they confront the truth. They realize it can reflect on them only if they refuse it. In both cases, victim-perpetrator bonds are broken.

In the U.S., where I live and practice, essentially everyone comes from a lineage of immigration—though how recently those journeys took place varies widely. I work with people who embody the spectrum of immigration stories: people who are immigrants, people who are first-generation Americans, and people whose ancestors have been here for multiple generations. And, of course, many of my clients' maternal and paternal lineages represent two completely distinct cultural inheritances that are sometimes at odds or, at the least, can be confusing to reconcile.

One of my clients, Mary, was a first-generation American whose white father was from Germany and whose Afro-Caribbean mother was from Guadeloupe. We would often conduct our sessions slipping back and forth between French and English without even noticing. Mary could also speak fluent German—a trilingual whiz kid, like so many children of immigrants. Her parents met at Columbia University in the early 1980s, fell in love while attending anti-apartheid protests, and decided to stay in New York City—rather than settle in either Germany or Guadeloupe—where they felt their soon-to-arrive biracial child would have the best chance of fitting in and the greatest opportunities. Mary had grown up independent and confident, a true New York

City kid taking the subway solo by 11, with friends from all over the world. Much of her mother's family had moved to the city over the course of her childhood, and she spent the summers in Germany with her beloved grandparents. She felt deeply connected to both sides of her family, as well as to her own Blackness within American culture, which was markedly different from her mother's French-inflected Caribbean identity. When I met Mary, she was in her thirties and had been a successful artist for more than a decade, with major gallery representation.

But the day Mary showed up in my office, she hadn't painted a new work for almost a year. She was in crisis, a potentially career-ending creative dry spell. I soon learned that Mary's paternal grandfather, with whom she had been especially close, had died just over a year earlier and Mary was still grieving him. But Mary's grief was complicated. During her stay in Germany for her grandfather's funeral, it had come to light that he had been a member of the Hitler Youth. Growing up, Mary had asked her dad about the war and about her grandparents' lives during wartime. "Were Opa and Oma Nazis?" she had once asked in fear when her middle school class took a field trip to the Museum of Jewish Heritage (the museum is "A Living Memorial to the Holocaust"). "What?! No," her father had said. "They were just regular people, and they were too young to fight in the war." That was it—they had never really talked about the Holocaust again. Mary didn't think much of it. After all, her father was married to a Black woman and had a Black child. Her grandparents *adored* her.

But the revelation about her grandfather threw into turmoil everything she thought she knew about him—and about herself. Had her grandfather actually been a white supremacist this whole time? Had *his* parents played an active role in the murder of millions of people? What had he really thought of her? She couldn't ask him, of course, and her grandmother was no longer alive either. Her father professed total ignorance. She felt deeply ashamed. For the first time, she felt self-conscious of her Germanness; previously she had thought of it as separate from her—her father had transmitted his whiteness to her, but *she* was American. Now she felt stained, culpable, complicit. She stopped speaking German with her father and extended family. She began compulsively telling her Jewish friends about her grandfather. It was weird and awkward, she told me. Her friends seemed confused and irritated with her, as if she were asking them for something. One of them, a close girlfriend, said, "I'm not sure what you want from me. Am I supposed to grant you absolution?" Mary didn't know. Worse than anything, she felt like an impostor who didn't have a right to lay claim to her Blackness. Her ancestors, enslaved, had worked sugar cane plantations on Guadeloupe. Though she was biracial, Mary had always taken comfort in the fact that none of her white ancestors had owned slaves. They weren't even French. They had been hanging out in Bavaria minding their own business; they weren't the "bad guys." But they were bad guys. And she loved them.

In the past, Mary had always turned to her art to navigate the difficult passages in life. Through her art, she made sense of herself and of the world. She started reading obsessively about the Holocaust and about the history of slavery in Guadeloupe. She tried to paint her way to reconciliation, but the paintings felt forced, belabored, and unnatural. She couldn't make sense of anything and she couldn't paint. She stopped speaking with her father and stopped visiting her parents, who had moved to upstate New York. She stopped returning the calls of her gallerist.

Mary and I began working on acknowledging what is. This was especially critical for Mary because she would never have "answers." She would never know the "truth" about her grandfather. All she had were facts. Her grandfather had been a member of the Hitler Youth. He had never spoken of the war that she could remember. He had unequivocally loved her. In fact, she had felt that he understood her and accepted her better than anyone in her family. It was he who had encouraged her to pursue her art. She had to consent to that reality—all of it, including how much she loved him. In a constellation, we had Mary extend her hand to her grandfather and welcome him back into place. "I will never know your story," she told his representative. "I accept your love as it is."

As Mary became comfortable acknowledging what is, she began speaking with her dad again, who acknowledged that he had intentionally avoided asking his parents about the war. He hadn't wanted to know. On a visit upstate, Mary had a startling conversation with her mom. While Mary talked with her about what she'd been going through, her mother took her hand and said, "But Mary, of course there is some French blood in us," and haltingly shared with her some of the "women's stories" passed down from mother to daughter that her grandmother had shared with her, about the relationships between their matriarchs and French owners. "I didn't like to think about it," Mary's mother told her. Mary realized her parents had kept her naive on purpose; they were deeply uncomfortable with parts of their family histories themselves and wanted to protect Mary. She saw how their desire to shelter her had made her a sheltered person: how despite being an artist, she was strangely incurious about politics, about travel (beyond her visits to Germany and Guadeloupe), about life outside of New York City in general, and about her own privilege as the daughter of two well-regarded lawyers. Curiosity had been anathema to protecting themselves, and Mary, from the painful parts of their legacy.

As Mary's ability to honor and respect the fates of her ancestors grew, her curiosity bloomed alongside it and her creativity returned in full flower. She moved away from the commercially successful but somewhat anodyne landscapes she had painted previously and gravitated toward more challenging abstract work that secured her the critical appreciation for which she had always longed. After one of her last sessions, done remotely, Mary asked me if I wanted a studio tour. As she panned her camera around the light-filled space, I saw what looked like a small altar in the corner, laid with eucalyptus, surrounding a small black-and-white photo of a young boy. "That's him," Mary said, "my grandfather." For many of my clients, the personal issues that led them to work with me reflect dynamics and entanglements that emerge from the impact of immigration on their family system. At the root of their pain (and the disorder in their family system) are issues of divided identity, loyalty, sacrifice, duty, allegiance, and, of course, belonging. The entire concept of belonging is even more fraught in such contexts.

When I met my client Tristan, he was living in New York City temporarily due to his wife's job. Tristan had lived in London since he was six years old (he was 29 when we met), but he was originally from Croatia. A year into the Croatian War of Independence, his mother had fled with him and his siblings to England, while his father had stayed behind to fight the Yugoslav Army. Even as an adult, Tristan still had vivid dreams of bombings and gunfire. Though his father had survived the war, their three-year separation had been deeply traumatic to Tristan. As a six-year-old, he had felt abandoned. After the war, his father was different too. "Part of him was missing. He would sort of zone out at times," Tristan said. "I missed my 'real' daddy and wondered when he would come back."

Once the family was reunited, they settled permanently in London. During school holidays, they would visit family in Croatia, but they never lived there again. Still, despite more than two decades in Great Britain, Tristan felt like an outsider there. When I asked him if he would feel more comfortable in Croatia, he said no, "it's my homeland, but it isn't my home."

The one place Tristan did feel at home was with his wife, who happened to be six years older than he was. At 35, she felt it was now or never to start trying for a baby. Tristan had come to me because although before getting married he had told his wife he wanted kids, he had been resisting taking the steps to get her pregnant. The clock was ticking, but Tristan now felt overwhelmingly unready to be a father. He sought me out hoping to resolve his resistance to parenthood since he loved his wife deeply and didn't want to lose his marriage.

Tristan felt rootless, so he was struggling with how to put down roots, how to have a family of his own. And he was grappling with what he could receive, as a man, from his country of origin and from his father. The two were deeply interlinked for him, a tangle of violence and sadness. Though his father had always been kind and gentle with his children, Tristan knew he'd been a soldier and that he had likely killed people. The war itself had ravaged Tristan's hometown, leveling buildings and leaving mounds of rubble behind. It became clear that for Tristan "home" and "father" were both subconsciously associated with destruction. He had resisted making London home both as a legacy of his parents' nationalism and out of his inner child's fear that doing so would lead to the destruction of his home. He was also uncomfortable with his own masculinity, which he associated with fighting; he was terrified of his rage and anger and his power as a man.

Together we worked on healing Tristan's inner child and answering the question "How can I receive from my country of origin?" In constellation, Tristan reconciled himself to his father's abandonment and his absence after he returned. He offered his father a secure place of belonging, exactly as he was. He practiced telling his father, "I welcome you home, Dad" and "You are my father, exactly as you are. You sacrificed part of yourself to secure safety and freedom for us." He practiced talking to his "little boy," telling him, "You have nothing to fear. The war is over. Daddy is fine. I will take care of you now." He began engaging with the positive, productive nature of the masculine, meditating on its healthy aspects, such as guiding, adventurousness, energy, structure, and commitment.

On their next vacation, Tristan brought his wife to Croatia, which he had never done before. He introduced her to his extended family. They traveled through the country, experiencing its beauty. They spent three weeks there; it was the longest Tristan had visited the country in adulthood, and the longest amount of time he'd spoken Croatian almost exclusively since he'd been six. On their way back to New York, they stopped in London to see friends and family. While they were there, Tristan planted a small tree in the yard of their home that he'd brought from Croatia. Back in New York, Tristan and his wife learned she was pregnant.

A bit into her second trimester, she and Tristan moved back to London. About five months after that, Tristan let me know that he and his wife had welcomed a baby boy. They had decided to buy a summer home in Croatia and raise their children bilingual. It was beautiful to witness Tristan's healing and joy.

Applying a systemic view to our family's larger immigration narratives (i.e., their stories not only about their journeys but about the cultures and countries from which they came) can help us better identify the dynamics within an individual family system, how our entanglements reflect an imbalance not only in our family system but also in our family's relationship to the larger system(s) in which it exists. When we honor our ancestors, we can then access our identity on our own terms.

The silent impact that our roots can have on our behaviors can be a big surprise. Our cultures and larger cultural histories often set the foundation for our family systems. In Europe, where there is more homogeneity and relationship between national identity and ethnicity (though this is and has been rapidly changing since the postwar period), entanglements often emerge from dynamics that are deeply culturally rooted: Through the work of Hellinger and other facilitators, some clear patterns in Family Constellations have been noted in relationship to national identities. In Italy, the centrality of the "mama" often creates intimacy and bonding issues in heterosexual relationships; in Germany, guilt and perpetrator anxiety tied to the Holocaust have been seen to play a part in depression issues; in Norway, "sailor stories" (absent fathers out at sea, mothers taking care of family) are often behind addiction struggles, rooted in a sense of masculine "uselessness"; in Ireland, mass emigration that created "living ghosts" of family members led to many family system exclusions and entanglements. Of course, every family is unique. Just because you come from a certain background doesn't mean its prevalent dynamics will impact your family.

For some of my clients, religion plays a powerful and sometimes toxic role in their family system. As a result, their identity is often bound to rejecting the religion, consuming any energy they might otherwise have to dedicate to exploring what does sustain them at the soul level. When they are able to truly acknowledge what is regarding how their family practiced its religious traditions—to accept and agree to that reality and reinclude that aspect of the family system in their sense of identity— their energy is no longer consumed in fighting it. They are freed from its bindings and liberated to explore and even connect to spirituality as they wish.

In my own healing process, the ability to recognize patterns not only within my family system but also in the larger forces at work (particular to the countries and histories within which my family system resided) added a deeper, additional layer to my ability to acknowledge what is. Over time, not only could I see that the fates of my ancestors belonged to them and respect that, I could truly, fully grasp the ways in which those fates were the product of even greater systems. This made it easier to occupy a place of suspended moral judgment so that I could welcome back into my system those I had excluded.

The story of my father and his family had always been a bit of a mystery to me. I knew he'd been born in Limoges, France, to my French grandmother, but that my grandfather had not been French; he'd been German and Prussian. And I knew that my grandfather had abandoned my grandmother when my father was an infant, disappearing when my father was just two months old. My father would eventually meet his father for the first time at 27, but following that initial meeting they'd had no relationship. I myself had never met my grandfather. Later, I would learn that it was my father who chose to remain estranged from his father, even rejecting my grandfather's offer to deed him family land.

Of course, in leaving us, my father ended up doing to his children exactly what had been done to him. He repeated the pattern of his first, most profound rejection of abandonment by his father, carrying this forward in the system from inheritance to legacy. Interestingly, my father waited until we were in our twenties to cut contact with us, the age at which he had been when his father attempted reconciliation.

As I immersed myself in Family Constellations, I was able to come to terms with the way in which my father was entangled in a dynamic with his father—how he had taken up his father's fate, initially trying to "correct" it through his own marriage and fatherhood but eventually being drawn to fill his absent father's place in the system. This understanding was enough for me to set down the burden of the story I'd been carrying (that I wasn't deserving of my father's love) and disrupt my own pattern of seeking partners who confirmed this narrative (that I wasn't worthy of any man's love).

In 2013, after a lot of work on my relationship with my father through Family Constellations, I had the urge to write him a letter. Though I was still uncertain about the possibility of ever reconciling with him, I wanted closure on my end. As I was finally able to understand why he had estranged himself (or, to be more precise, as I was finally able to understand that the estrangement was not my fault), I reached out, outlining my hopes and love for our relationship, which otherwise always seemed to get lost in misunderstandings. Two years later, in 2015, my father and I reunited in New York City. The four days we spent together were full of peace and acceptance. We did not talk about the past; we focused only on the present moment and this new chance to create a balanced relationship.

Over time, this created the space for me to ask him all the questions I'd had about his family—the questions that I'd always sensed were too fraught to broach growing up, and that later I'd wanted to ask from a place of blame and accusation (i.e., I was looking for the answer to "Why are you hurting me?"), which shut my father down. After our reconciliation, my motives were more neutral; they stemmed from curiosity and intellectual hunger to better understand our family system. And my dad seemed to sense this, answering me in a way he never had before. But what I learned proved to offer an unexpectedly new path to even deeper healing.

Though both my parents are French, my father's side of the family was not French. My grandfather had been born in Munich, but his parents were not German, exactly—they were Prussian. Prussia, of course, no longer exists. The hugely powerful state once covered much of what is Germany today (all but Southern Germany) and large swaths of Poland. But by the end of World War II, its existence was essentially erased. Seeing the writing on the wall and fearing what was to come (as well as not supporting Nazism), my great-grandparents left Europe just before the war and immigrated to Argentina. Unfortunately, they left my grandfather behind at the boarding school he was attending in Limoges, taking only his little sister with them. They meant to return for him at the end of the school year, but the outbreak of the war prevented that, essentially orphaning him in France for the next four years—until he was conscripted into the French Army, then captured and held as a prisoner of war by the Russians.

When the war was over and he was liberated, my grandfather returned to Limoges, the only home he'd known for the last part of his life. There, he met my grandmother and they conceived, "out of wedlock," as the saying used to go, my father. At the same time, my grandfather's parents in Argentina were finally able to send for him. They did not want to return to Europe. The homeland they had known was literally gone, and postwar Germany was in a state of ruin. Though my grandfather asked my grandmother to marry him and move to Argentina, she did not want to leave her family or her country behind, especially after enduring so much calamity and upheaval in the war. My grandfather, perhaps longing to end his own "orphaning," chose to go to Argentina without her—or his newborn son.

Learning all of this broke my heart a little, but it also brought me greater peace, as it deepened my empathy for my ancestors, just humans like me, caught in the inexorable forces of politics and war, and struggling with difficult fates and limited choices in the face of such fates. Here were people whose lives were shaped by exile, by erasure, by orphaning, by immigration, by the loss of home and identity—literally and figuratively—at every turn. I could see how these historical dynamics seeded our family system with a sense of displacement, of being forever not at home in the world, and of desperately searching for that home, sometimes to our own detriment and the detriment of those we loved. And I could see that my own urgent need to leave France in my twenties (though I loved Paris, where I'd grown up, and Brittany, where I'd spent countless summers and holidays) was a part of this rootlessness. Even in the U.S., I had already moved from Miami to California, back to Miami, and then to New York, still searching for that feeling of being in the right place. In confronting this entanglement with history, I was able, at last, to extricate myself from it—to settle within myself, to recognize that I made my home.

And in honoring the fate of my ancestors fully, I was able to draw strength from them, from their history. Despite the choices they had made (or because of them), they had still endured, and I was here. Honoring their journey—and its peripatetic nature— was incredibly helpful in keeping me grounded as I was staying in friends' homes and searching for a new apartment through the many long months of 2020, as the pandemic ravaged New York City and the globe. For six months, I struggled with fear as I relied on the largesse of friends, but I never gave up hope or lost sight of the big picture, because I knew I would find my home when the time was right.

Honoring our ancestors by including them in our family systems, respecting their fates, and leaving their responsibilities to them helps us to make peace not only with our past but also with the complexities of history and culture. We are reminded that we belong to a family system, and that that system belongs in turn to a wider web of intersecting systems. When we can really keep this truth in mind, we are reminded of our deep interconnectedness, not just within our families but across humanity.

We need this remembering now more than ever. When we practice awareness of our interconnections, we become more conscious of the quality of our connections. We are more open to the truth of our shared responsibility to each other when it comes to our experiences as individuals, which are ultimately inseparable from the collective.

The coronavirus pandemic, for most of us our first truly global experience, laid bare how deeply interconnected we are, how our individual actions ripple across our communities, and how our mutual well-being relies on each of us taking accountability and responsibility for our choices. At the same time, that increasing consciousness of our shared humanity opened more people's eyes to the injustices that were always there in plain sight. Finally people from all walks of life were unwilling to look away from the institutionally sanctioned murders of people like George Floyd and Breonna Taylor, joining in—often for the first time—the critical and inspiring civil rights movement Black Lives Matter, rejecting racism and actively working to become anti-racist, from the personal level to the highest levels of our governments and institutions.

We are living at an inflection point, a cultural and historic crossroads of great urgency. As we grapple daily with extreme political partisanship, racism, and xenophobia, the threats of climate change, the rise in gun violence, and the sometimes painful reverberations of our shared histories, we are hungrier than ever to connect authentically, to affirm our shared humanity, to explore the roots of our identity, and to heal our pasts so that we can create a new vision of the future, one that is inclusive and uplifting for all.

Taking a systemic view can help us achieve and sustain these ambitions. We begin with ourselves. And as we do the work and build the muscle, we connect not only with our authenticity and power to determine our own stories but also with the power of seeing others within the greater context of the systems they inhabit. We are rewarded with a more complex, wide, and deep view of others' lives, as well as our own. In accepting the richness of life, accepting rather than resisting its complexity, life itself becomes less narrow and the possibilities open to all of us become so much greater.

AFFIRMATIONS

I honor my ancestors' fates even as I write my own destiny.

I accept the blessings of my country's past, the challenges and the pain, and will carry those blessings with me.

By knowing the history of my country,
I can be a messenger for the next generation.

EXERCISE: Honoring Your Ancestors

Do you know where your ancestors were from? Honoring our ancestors means honoring their experiences, which were shaped by their cultures and histories. Honoring the culture, countries, and histories of your ancestors is not about cosplaying as an Irish person on Saint Patrick's Day. It is about bearing witness to lives lived and about sharing and celebrating their legacies through food, art, music, language, and stories, including the difficult ones. If you don't know where your ancestors were from, start by asking relatives if you are able to do so. If you don't have family who can fill in the blanks, you may consider using a service like 23andMe or Ancestry.com. Once you do know (or if you knew already), see if you can trace the path from there to where you are now. You can do this through oral tradition, shared testimony, and interviews with experts, or just by discussing it with someone who shares a similar background with you. In other words, listen to stories passed down through your family, talk to an elder, speak with an academic, take a friend to lunch who has more access to genealogy and ask them what they've learned. Seek out recipes from your culture and prepare them (or visit a restaurant that specializes in the foods of that culture, if you're lucky enough to have one nearby); ask a parent or grandparent to teach you how to cook a specific dish. Read the folktales and literature of the culture. Take a language class or learn some basic phrases via an app like Duolingo. If you're able, record your elderly relatives talking about their families. There may even be a museum where you live dedicated to documenting your cultural inheritance. Visit it! And celebrate contemporary iterations of your cultural inheritance: artists who share your identity or identities and who explore it, explicitly or implicitly, in their work. Celebrate the best of the past in yourself.

Create an altar for your ancestors. This could be on a small table, on a shelf, or on a mantle—any surface you have cleared and dedicated to this purpose. If you have photos of your ancestors, place them on the altar. If you do not have photos of them, feel free to use representative images such as historical photos of members of your culture. Light candles for them. Place a flower in a vase near the photos. Ask your ancestors for wisdom. Call on your ancestors for guidance and protection. Tell your children stories about your lineage. Keep the chain of wisdom alive. We are all connected in an intricate, intimate web. The more we remember our place in this web—and that we're not isolated entities—the stronger we will be.

CHAPTER 2

Belonging, Order, and Entanglement

D o you ever feel that no matter how much you try—to change your habits, your limiting beliefs, your self-sabotaging behaviors—that you remain stuck, or quickly drawn back to your old ways, even as you recognize them as obstacles to your happiness? Do you feel unfulfilled, a nagging sense that you should be on a different path, but not why or what that path might be? It's likely you're caught in an **entanglement**, an energetic connection with a family member of a previous generation that is constricting your growth and freedom.

Always hold close to your heart the core truth of Family Constellations: *It did not start with me.* It's never truer than when we pause to explore how we came to unconsciously identify and become entangled with those who came before us—whether we know them or not. Family Constellations reveals, in particular, the surprising hold the dead have on the living, and the ways that traumas are transmitted down through generations—the forceful impact on our present of pasts we've never experienced. Put simply, the lives of those who have come before you (both dead and still living), some of whom you may have never known, can and do actively shape your life as you live it now.

I know, this is difficult to fully wrap our minds around. But remember two of those cardinal rules that govern the family system, *belonging* and *order*? Everyone born into a family, past or present, has a right to belong to it. And all of the members of a family have the *same* right to belong to it. Everyone has a place, or an order, in their family system. Everyone has the right to be part of a lineage. That's the gift of belonging.

The problem is, when a family member is denied belonging, be it through exclusion or because they have been concealed, forgotten, or gone unmourned, the family system is thrown out of order. A missing family member is like a tear in the fabric of the system. The family system will seek to repair that tear by replacing the missing member with someone of a subsequent generation, creating an *entanglement*. Unfortunately, entanglement doesn't restore order, it only deepens the damage to the family system. In an entanglement, you take the place of another person. *You're no longer fully committed to your own life*—you are simultaneously living another's destiny on their behalf. You are identified with the fate of another. At best this leads to being stuck and unfulfilled; at worst, it repeats a cycle, renews the pattern, reproducing hurts and pain that didn't start with you, but the burden of which you are now carrying.

And speaking of hurt and pain: Family systems also become disordered by traumatic events experienced by family members, such as illness, death, or violence and all they encompass, in complex ways. Untreated, a wound to an individual also wounds the family system. When a family member is caught in the trauma, when a person cannot let go of grief or relinquish their identity as a victim, for example, they cannot fully occupy their rightful place in the family system. They are paralyzed in time, their destiny stymied. The energy of the family system, which ideally flows forward in time, is obstructed there. So, as always, the family system seeks to repair itself, to restore order, drawing a later family member to "fix" what should have been, or to act for or atone for that person (as opposed to replacing that person). In this way, you may become unknowingly identified with members of your family. And in this way, the family system transmits our traumas, our losses, our grievances from one generation to the next. Entanglement, again.

Entanglements prevent us from living fully and wholly because they prevent us from pursuing the path of our own destiny. In a sense, they create a divided loyalty of the self. They trap us in the past, which goes counter to the flow of life. When you are busy trying to live out the life of another, to compensate for their loss or correct a traumatic event, your own organic needs, curiosities, passions, hurts, and gifts become harder to see, hear, and feel clearly. When you disentangle yourself from these knotty and too-often-invisible dynamics, you are liberated to finally recognize and pursue your own highest calling in service to your highest self.

Furthermore, when you disentangle yourself from the destiny of another family member, you are simultaneously working to restore order to the family system, both healing the past (where the disorder in the system originated) and preventing future entanglements. There's so much beauty in that. Family Constellations empowers us not only to heal ourselves but also to nurture and care for our ancestors, as well as those who will come after us. *You* can break the cycle of estrangement, of trauma, of destinies unfulfilled. *You* can reconcile the past and the present, so that your future is one entirely of your own making. All you need to do is take one small, intentional step toward your destiny, toward breaking any entanglements that are tethering you to a life that isn't your own. And the first step to breaking an entanglement is simply to learn its signs. Are you ready?

EXERCISE:

"It Did Not Start with Me"—Learning the Signs of Entanglement

Freeing yourself from an entanglement and restoring order to your family system begins with *knowing* you're entangled. But how do you know if you might be entangled with a family member? The first step is recognizing the signs of entanglement. For this exercise, you'll need a notebook or a journal (a digital document works too) in which to answer the prompts that follow, and some quiet, uninterrupted time. Our goal here is to give you the space to pause and explore whether you could be feeling like, behaving like, suffering like, atoning for, or carrying the grief of someone who came before you. For the sake of clarity, I think it's best to answer each question on a separate page of your notebook or notepad. The exercise works best if you answer the questions in the order given. If there are questions to which you don't know the answers, that's okay. These questions are designed to get you *attuned* to the signs of entanglement; sometimes that's all you need to do to begin unraveling one.

Please note, Family Constellations asserts that we are at the center of a family system that produces impact over seven generations: three before us, our current generation, and three after us. (Of course, this links us even further back to our ancestors, and forward in time to our descendants.) So for the questions that follow, when you are reflecting on family members who have come before you, focus on the families of your parents, your grandparents, and your great-grandparents.

You may also have limited means of addressing these questions, and that's okay too. For different reasons, from estrangement to immigration to adoption, among others, many of us may not be able to put together a record of key dates in our families or seek out the stories of our ancestors. Regardless, *you always have a narrative*, even if that narrative is "I don't know." "I don't know" is a story, too, an equally valid and powerful one. Just remember: It did not start with you. Whatever you cannot resolve in your present moment, give it back to your past; give it back to your ancestors.

Finally, I'd like to draw your attention to the fact that many of the questions that follow operate in a framework of guilt, shame, rejection, anger, or silence. This is because entanglements emerge from the (often unresolved) *feelings* about an event, action, or person, not from the event, action, or person itself. A family member whose death is mourned and whose life is celebrated is unlikely to feel unseen and unheard; they belong to the family system, and so an entanglement with them is unlikely. Similarly, a person may experience a trauma but feel supported in its aftermath (personally, socially, legally, therapeutically, etc.). In such a case, that trauma is unlikely to cause an entanglement with a family member in the next generation.

- Do you ever feel that you're not in charge of your life? Are you unhappy in your work or with your relationships, despite them seeming "good on paper"? Do you experience financial instability despite your best efforts to be secure? Do you feel that you've worked intensely on your issues but they continue to persist?

- Do you regularly experience emotions or routinely engage in/avoid behaviors that are difficult to explain in the context of your life experience? Do you have any irrational fears? Feeling regularly overwhelmed or blocked by persistent emotions is a sign that those emotions may be transgenerational, as is engaging in or avoiding certain behaviors. (It may be helpful to think about this as compulsions and phobias.) What are those fears or emotions? When do you experience them? When did you start experiencing them? Take time to write through this, doing your best to answer as a neutral observer of your life, with as little judgment as possible.

- Do you know of any family members who were rejected by or are/were estranged from the family? If so, who? Note their name and their relationship to you (e.g., "Lydia, great-aunt, my paternal grandmother's older sister"). Why were they rejected? Note the reason, regardless of its validity, and without judgment (e.g., pregnancy out of wedlock, marriage to an "unacceptable" spouse, sexuality, leaving a religion, criminal or violent acts).

- Do you know of any traumas in the family that, for the most part, the family does not discuss because the event or events were too painful, shameful, or terrible to talk about (e.g., parental abandonment, adoption of a child out of the family, rape, suicide, accidents, crimes, deaths of family members)? What was the trauma? To whom did it happen? Again, note as much as you know about the event, as well as the name and relationship of the family member to whom it happened.

- Are there any family members for whom guilt or pain has prevented them from grieving the loss of another family member? Who? Why? Note the name of the unmourned or unacknowledged family member, their relation to you, and how they died.

- Are there any defining generational traumas in your family, i.e., experiences such as immigration, living as refugees, war, genocide, poverty? What are or were they? In which generation did they have primary impact? Write down as much as you know. What stories have you been told and by whom? What *don't* you know? Sometimes what is left out is more revealing than what is included.

Whew! That was a lot of work. Give yourself a hand (and perhaps a glass of wine or a hot bath). It's not easy engaging with some of the tougher aspects of our family histories, but it is a wonderful adventure to truly know where you came from. My only recommendation is that when that discovery process is no longer enjoyable, please let it be. This means your work is done and that you know everything you are meant to know. It's always important to know when to start and when to finish. (Though everything you've just done here will be the foundation for the rest of the chapter, so you'll want to keep what you wrote close at hand as you continue to read.)

The Call of Ghosts

Absent family members—missing people—hold tremendous energy in our family systems. They haunt us. When we fail to acknowledge or mourn a loss, when we try to erase, silence, or forget family members whose deaths, or whose actions in life, have been painful or shameful, we will find that they insist upon being seen and heard—and the harder the family system will work to return itself to order (the state in which every family member is in his or her ordained place) via entanglement.

Who is an absent family member? An absent family member is a person who no longer occupies his or her place within the family system; they have left (purposefully or inadvertently) or been cast out or, often, both. They can be living or dead (through Family Constellations, we see that the border between the realm of the living and the realm of the dead is far more porous than we might have thought). Yet it's not enough that a person leaves us, literally or figuratively—it's how family members feel about that loss that creates entanglement. When our shame or grief causes us to exclude a family member from the family system, their right to belong is denied.

Because we live in the context of a shared culture with shared values (though those values are changing over time), there are certain categories of loss that tend to lead toward more grief or shame. There are events you can look to for clues about any absent people within your own family: Instances of early death, abortion, miscarriage, childbirth, terminal illness, or suicide can all point to a missing person and a source of entanglement.

Think about your own family. Is there a child who died early, a topic so painful that no one spoke of him or her? A great-grandparent who lost the family fortune, relegating his children to penury, rejected in death as the source of family misfortune (quite literally)? Or perhaps a parent who abdicated his or her responsibility, leading the other parent to strike them from the record, as it were?

This is a good moment to review and think about your answer to the question regarding deaths in your family that other family members avoid discussing. Guilt and overwhelming grief around a death can point to a family member who's right to belong has been essentially denied—and to an entanglement with the deceased. Generally, when a person is entangled with an estranged or deceased person, he or she unconsciously takes over the fate of this absent member of the family and lives it out. You might find yourself caught in toxic and repetitive behaviors you know are harmful but that you cannot seem to stop or avoid; you are driven to repair something that does not belong to you.

For example, do you regularly put yourself in danger or engage in any kind of extreme or compulsive behavior? Although having a few tattoos—even quite a few—is well within normal bounds culturally, a desire to cover the body in tattoos (especially the face) could be a sign that you're not at home in your skin, for example. That desire to erase the self or transform can point to an entanglement. You might take a look at previous family generations to see if anyone died in a dramatic way or at a young age. If so, you might resonate with the event or pattern immediately. Consider any way in which you might be connected with the deceased person or exhibit any similar patterns—shared interests, physical traits, names, illnesses, life events, professions, odd coincidences.

An entanglement may exhibit in a primarily emotional rather than behavioral mode. One of my clients came to me because she had an overpowering fear of death. She could not stop thinking about dying. It was becoming problematic—she was having trouble getting out of bed every day. You could say she was no longer fully living. We did a one-on-one constellation using paper footprints as representatives. After carefully arraying the members of her family, she was drawn to stand in the place of her great-aunt. "I feel at home here," she said, certain but also surprised. The entanglement was clear. Quickly I learned that her great-aunt had died at age four in a house fire. The little girl's fear and sense of abandonment was palpable in the room.

Though my client had known the bare facts of her great-aunt's death, she had never made the connection between it and her fear of dying. Even though her own mother was afraid of fire, as was she, she had never recognized the pattern echoing through time. She rarely, if ever, thought of her great-aunt—it was just a story, though sad, of something tragic that happened long ago to a child she had never known. Like her parents before her, her grandmother almost never spoke of her lost little sister; the horror and pain of her story was too much to bear. Her great-aunt was an absent person, excluded from the family system because the horror of her death was too unbearable. As long as no one recognized her, a new family member would be drawn to fill her place. Of course, my client knew about her great-aunt—just like most of us have some sense of our family's losses, even as we look away from them. In a constellation, the power of the knowing field reveals what we've been unable to see clearly. But this power is accessible to you now, in this moment, by pausing and looking for that invisible thread that links one generation to the next.

Sometimes in an entanglement, we may not necessarily engage in dangerous behavior but rather resist behaviors we unknowingly perceive as dangerous in an attempt to atone for the fate of a deceased family member. When we preemptively avoid certain experiences as a defense mechanism, we are prescribing the boundaries of our lives, making them smaller. Think about it: Have you ever avoided something you may have wanted, such as a relationship, out of fear of getting hurt? You were protecting yourself, yes, but weren't you also missing out on joy and growth? In one constellation I had the privilege of participating in, a young woman was hoping to resolve her intimacy issues with her husband; though she loved him and was attracted to him, she never felt like having sex. The field revealed that her great-grandmother, who died in childbirth, had not been recognized and her representative felt unseen. Her widower rarely spoke of her. The surviving children grew up knowing very little about their mother. Her grandmother, in turn, nearly died in childbirth. And her mother had been diagnosed with ovarian cancer—one of the rarer and more lethal cancers. It turned out that this young woman, the great-granddaughter, was entangled with her great-grandmother. She had a deep fear of motherhood and childbirth, and a resistance to becoming pregnant. Her lack of desire was not rooted in her relationship.

In both cases, my clients were able to come into awareness of an entanglement. But more than that, they were able to free themselves of the entanglement while restoring order to their family systems—by healing the wounds of the past. How? Through *acknowledging* their ancestors and *welcoming* them back into a state of belonging. My client spoke to her great-aunt, recognizing her death and the fear she must have experienced, while also reasserting her independent identity, using language you can use, as well: "I give you a place in my family. It happened to you, not me. I break free from that fear." A year later, she was no longer afraid of dying. She not only got out of bed every day, but she also had ended up writing a book.

My client who had come to me struggling with intimacy was also able to disentangle herself from the destiny of her great-grandmother and set that energy at peace. The participant who took the role of the great-grandmother in that constellation had been lying on the floor, waiting to be acknowledged. When my client knelt and took her hand, recognizing her pain and death and welcoming her back into her rightful place in the family system, she felt lighter. A few months later, she sent me an e-mail letting me know that she was expecting her first child.

It's been my honor to be part of several constellations in which absent family members are just waiting to be recognized. Often the dead are actually standing, waiting for permission to finally lie down and be at peace. (It's exhausting to stand while dead, and the same goes for the living lying on the floor—it's exhausting to pretend to be dead while you are alive.) Each time this has happened organically and been instantly recognizable, as the members of the family constellation look down in sync, searching, asking themselves, *Who am I looking for? Who is missing?*

In all of these constellations, many tears flowed. In each one, the energy was very intense and even draining, but at the end of the constellations, as the resolution unfolded, we experienced a new flow of serenity and release in the room. They were breathtaking, beautiful, and respectful ceremonies of acknowl-edgment and inclusion for the people waiting to be recognized and accepted as members of the family system.

Acknowledging the missing can be more difficult when the source of their absence is shameful, however. As we've seen, shame plays an especially large part in deepening the exclusion of many people who are absent from their family systems. Violent deaths and suicides cause some of the most powerful entanglements; not only are the deceased wrenched from the family system, but their deaths often go silenced out of overpowering grief, fear, or shame among the surviving family. But missing people need to be accepted, recognized, and loved no matter what destiny they chose to live. You must acknowledge their right to be part of the family system, regardless of the difficulty of their destiny. By respecting their destiny, you respect the order in your family system. Doing so will release the heavy weight of secrets and, accordingly, the unconscious desire to atone for someone or to balance the system through suicide, self-harm, or other dangerous or stuck behaviors.

Doing so does not mean *approving* of the destiny but rather accepting its reality (i.e., accepting the fact that it happened and no longer trying to avoid or conceal it) and therefore making room for the family member within the system once again. In an entanglement, you can do this by first recognizing the entan-glement, and by surrendering your attempt to live in that family member's place. This means understanding that the past cannot be unwritten, and owning *your* life. It means taking responsibility for your destiny—and for refusing to keep secrets that perpetuate a cycle of shame.

When we remove shame from our family stories, we can more readily reinclude missing members; we can put things in order. Indeed, when a secret is revealed by the person or people involved with it, it can powerfully impact the family system's well-being across the energetic level, as it did in my family. On Christmas Eve 2012, I was at my mother's house in Paris. My grandmother had died five months earlier, and it was already a bittersweet night— our first Christmas without her. As dinner drew to a close, my grandfather announced, out of the blue, that he had something to tell us. This was . . . well, weird. He is not a big talker, to put it mildly.

My grandfather proceeded to tell us that when he'd met my grandmother in late 1959, he'd actually been in a relationship with another woman, "Sabine," and that it had been serious—they'd discussed getting married. He lived in Paris at the time but had to travel to Brittany for work. While there, he met my grandmother and fell madly in love. He never went back to Paris. After a whirlwind courtship, my grandparents married in April 1960 and my mother was born early that December (yes, I've done the math).

My grandfather continued, somewhat haltingly. A few years earlier, he had found his former girlfriend online and reached out to her. By then, my grandmother was in the late stages of Alzheimer's disease. I think my grandfather must have been lonely and grieving, and accounting for his own mortality, though I'm not sure. Like I said, not a big talker. Despite the fact that my grandmother was the love of his life, he had never forgotten his girlfriend. She hadn't been his soul mate, but she had been the only other woman he'd loved. He had always wondered where she was and how she was doing, how her life had turned out.

They began corresponding and eventually met in person. Sabine revealed to him that she had been pregnant when they'd broken up—and that she had kept the baby, a little boy. He'd been born in the spring of 1960, just as my grandparents were marrying. Devastatingly, he had died at six months old, only months before the birth of my mother. Sabine had never remarried or had another child and had devoted the rest of her life to her career as a nurse.

My family sat in silence at the table. We had lived all our lives in ignorance of this child, who had been my grandfather's son, his first child, my mother's half brother, my lost uncle. The astonishing thing is that when my mother was a little girl, she used to ask her mother, "Where is my big brother?" My grandmother chalked this up to her daughter's curious mind and active imagination, and to the habit children have of measuring themselves against other families, always gently reminding her that she was their firstborn—there was no older brother. But my mother had always sensed an absence, and a peculiar grief shadowed her. Of course, though I would have to do a constellation for my mother, aunt, and uncle to identify any entanglements with their lost brother (no thank you), it has also been a theme of my uncle's life that he has always felt *rejected* and *unseen* by my grandfather.

A missing person does not need to cause an entanglement for their absence to be keenly felt and for a family system to be deeply affected. It is clear that my grandfather's son, and his first love, both of whom had "gone missing," had weighed heavily on our family system—on my grandfather and everyone who had radiated from him—because their return undeniably shifted our dynamic for the better. After that night, my grandfather became someone who no longer perceived feelings and sensitivity as a threat to his masculinity. He became someone who said, "I love you."

Some of us may know or sense that the version of the family history we have access to is not the full picture—that it contains dark spots, silences, secrets. As frustrating as it may be, often there is no way to uncover that secret, to learn its details. We might know the vague outlines of a relationship or an event or an incident (in other words, we know that something happened), but we'll never know the full story. Even though this can cause frustration and a fear that we're stuck in our entanglements, we all have an "emergency exit." It's accepting that sometimes *the secret is the story*. Accepting the secret, and the silence in which it lives, as a fact unto itself—acknowledging its existence and force—and releasing it to the past with love and respect, can also heal us. Endlessly seeking out the details can keep us in the past, in the sphere of the life that happened before us, and out of the light of clarity and the knowledge that we are responsible for our lives going forward.

When the dead have their place, they are peaceful, and they are finally experienced as a positive energy. Therefore, life flow energy, abundance, joy, and love come back into all the different generations. By taking care of our ancestors, we take care of our next generation. In Family Constellations, invisible forces are rendered visible, brought into the light. We are able to see and recognize them, tension is released, and instead of behaving unconsciously at their will, we move forward consciously. Belonging and order are restored to the family system. When the family system is in order, each member takes his or her rightful place—and in your rightful place, you are more at ease. This applies to every member of the family system and thus the family as a group, which begins to breathe easier. Love flows more freely.

AFFIRMATIONS

I see you and I give you a place in my heart.

I respect your fate and bow to your destiny,
and I honor you as my [family member].

I will hold on to the gift of life you have given me as long as I may; only when my time has come will I follow you.

EXERCISE: Recognition Ceremony—Restoring Order

Now that you've deepened your understanding of the effect of absent people in the family system and explored the possibility of absent people in your own family system, it's time to practice recognizing them, granting belonging, and restoring order—reconciling the pull of the past with our obligations to the present. A recognition ceremony for the absent person with whom you might be entangled can be a powerful way to restore their belonging and free you from the entanglement. If your journaling in the exercise "It Did Not Start with Me" didn't call to mind an absent family member, you can ask a family member (gently and with respect) about the possibility of any absent people in the family.

Even if you do not get answers that seem to help, I recommend that you still create a ceremony to recognize any missing people in your family. A recognition ceremony symbolizes both a return to belonging and a release from entanglement; it is important that the act signifies a welcome and a farewell. You can begin by addressing a letter to an absent or deceased family member. This should be an actual, physical letter. You can either write it by hand or type it out and then print it. Open the letter with, "I acknowledge you and I am letting you go . . ." Then, trust your heart and write whatever you want to share with this person. Close with, "I honor your fate. I recognize you as a member of my family, and I give you a place in my heart." Then again, let your heart speak for you. The only important thing is to feel very deeply inside of you: "I am doing this ceremony for you; now you can finally be at peace." Once you have written the letter, you can burn it or drop it in a mailbox. It is important that you do not keep the letter but rather that you let it go with respect (i.e., don't toss it in the trash can).

Echoing Patterns

Sometimes what haunts us is not the dead but the living and their unresolved grief and trauma, which they transmit through their children and their children's children—a sort of lineage of pain and loss. This creates an imbalance in the family system as powerful as belonging denied; it also entangles us in fates and destinies that are not our own.

When someone is entangled in the fate and destiny of another, sadly, they reproduce the imbalance that entangled them, as they are called to atone for parents or grandparents. When this happens, a pattern is created in the family dynamic, persistent and sneaky but visible if you choose to look for it. One of the simplest ways to illuminate such a pattern (and hopefully release it) in your own family is to review your answers to the exercise "It Did Not Start with Me." Label a sheet of paper or document "Patterns." Read through your answers carefully, first looking for *repeating names* and *unusual events* (an event in this context could mean early death, shared illnesses or disease, similar accidents, multiple marriages, episodes of immigration/emigration, etc.), making note of anything that emerges.

Shared names are common in many cultures, used to honor both the living and the dead. Though I respect the impulse here—honoring our loved ones and our ancestors *is* a generous and caring act—giving a child the same name as a family member, especially a deceased family member, could indicate an emerging entanglement or have an entangling impact on their life, connecting their fate in some way to the fate of the person they were named for. The namesake may remain in or repeat the same destiny (death at a similar age, for example) or fail to do so in a way that's equally painful. As far as I'm concerned, we already have so many things from our lineage to deal with, we don't need any more weight added to what we carry. A newborn is a new life, beginning, and cycle. Let's give him or her a chance to take the best part of their lineage and create something great from it with a fresh start. I strongly feel that if naming your child after a loved one is of importance to you that you either use the name as a middle name or that instead you choose a similar-sounding name or one that begins with the same letter (this is a common tradition among Ashkenazi Jewish families, for example).

If *you* are named after a deceased loved one, especially one who died early or tragically, don't shy away from your ancestor. Learn more about this part of your heritage, if you can. Recognize any tragic events that occurred, then separate yourself with love from any entanglements that you might have with the passed family member or child. First, recognize the earliest member of the family of whom you are aware that shared the name. Let's pretend for a moment that your name is Sasha and you know that you share the name with a great-grandfather. If you have a photo of him (or her), that's wonderful—you can hold the photo and, looking at it, state, "Sasha, I am your namesake. Thank you for sharing this piece of family identity with me." Next, recognize his or her life; you can say, "I acknowledge your life and thank you for my own. I would not be here without you." Finally, assert ownership of your own life; state, "I'm not here as a continuation/ extension of you. I'm here with my own life, and by living my life and embracing it, I will honor you. But I don't need to follow you or finish your unfinished business."

After looking for repeating or shared names and unusual events, review your notes for *key dates* and *ages*. These could be shared birthdays (or death days) or shared ages at which significant events occur across generations. For example, you and your uncle might share the same birthday. Or you and your great-grandmother might not share the same birthday, but perhaps at 31 she left behind her home country and at 31 you divorced— both events a kind of abandoning of an old way of life in search of a better future. Every family dynamic includes these key dates. The family tree exercise from Chapter 1 is also a powerful resource here, as are family members whom you might ask for more specifics about the timing of particular events in their past, such as war, miscarriages, suicides, or displacement (events that, unlike birth, death, or marriages, tend not to be noted on family trees), making note of how the timing may coincide with inflection points in your own life. These patterns can show us how we may be caught in entanglements that are part of a cycle of inherited trauma.

In my family, for example, trauma and tragedy appeared regularly at age 13—that strange moment on the cusp between childhood and adulthood when we crave independence but still seek the shelter of our parents. At 13, my paternal grandmother lost her grandfather and father on the same day, when they were shot on the platform of a train station at the height of World War II. Meanwhile, as mentioned earlier, my paternal grandfather was orphaned in his own way, also at age 13. His parents and sister were living in Argentina as WWII broke out, and when they were unable to retrieve him from France, where he was in boarding school, they left him behind. Eventually he was drafted into the war, only to become a Russian POW. After the war, he met my grandmother. When she became pregnant out of wedlock, he asked her to come to Argentina with him, but she chose to stay in

France. Growing up in 1950s small-town France as the child of an unwed mother was not easy for my father. He was bullied relentlessly for being the "son of a whore"—until, at age 13, he snapped and brutally attacked the boy who'd led the worst of it. And it was at 13 that I was sexually assaulted in London, on a trip my parents had sent me on to improve my fluency in English. Each of us was a child separated from our parents, forced to grow up before our time. We were stripped of our childhood, our lives sundered by innocence lost into a stark before and after.

As far as I've been able to tell, each one of us had been in the dark with this pattern of abandonment and trauma. I believe any one of us could—*can*, in my case—have broken the curse if only we'd been aware there was a pattern that needed acknowledging in the first place. Through the work of Family Constellations, I was able to shed light on that darkness and finally confront the depths of my own pain. Though I don't have children, it's my hope that if I do I'll have disrupted the pattern permanently—by taking responsibility for my shit so that no one in the next generation has to repair or fix it for me later—and that the worst that they will endure at 13 are the universal, everyday struggles of that awkward age. You have the same power, the power to disrupt a legacy of loss or violence. You are not a prisoner of what—or who—came before you, I promise. When you are able to see your life in the greater context of a family system, you can step back and more fully grasp the ways in which your ancestors are a source of power (both literal life energy and the wisdom of their accumulated experience) even as you harness that power to move forward in your own life consciously and with intent.

Voltaire wrote, "Each player must accept the cards life deals him or her. But once they are in hand, he or she alone must decide how to play the cards in order to win the game." The hand we are dealt is our fate—it is preordained, by the universe, by Source, by the divine, by genetics and history, whichever you are most comfortable with. The Latin word from which it comes, *fatum*, literally means "It has been spoken." It's already over and done with. The point is, we have no control over where or when or to whom we are born; that is our fate. It was my fate to be born in France in the late 20th century, to be born a woman, to be born to the parents I was. Our fates are inevitably connected to our ancestors. There is no us without them. But our destinies do not have to be. Our destinies are a result of how we play that hand—the choices we make on the paths we walk through our lives. Our fates are where we came from; our destinies are where we are going. What is your fate? What is your destiny?

When we are entangled with the fate of another person, we take on their destiny as our own and lose our way. When we recognize our entanglements, we have the power to preempt and disrupt old patterns, changing not only the course of our own lives—taking control of our destinies—but also the lives of those who come after us. Our family systems are in order, and each of us belongs where we are meant to be.

AFFIRMATIONS

I may share the same date of birth/name of my _____,
but I do not share his/her fate.

I have my own fate.

I belong to my family by living my own destiny.

EXERCISE:

Pattern Sorting—A Personal Inventory

At the start of this chapter, we began by looking to our family's past as a foundation for learning the signs of entanglement. Here, we reverse that order and begin with *your* past, taking a personal inventory of the critical events that have shaped you, as a tool for high-level pattern sorting. Once you have done so, use the inventory to structure a dialogue with willing family members.

If your grandparents are still alive, I encourage you to ask them if they would be open to filling in some of the details of their pasts with you. You can explain that you are looking to gain insight into formative events in the lives of family members to obtain a deeper understanding of the family history.

Being gentle with yourself as you do so, make a list of any important, traumatic, and/or significant events that have occurred in your life, starting from birth. Note your age at the time of each of those incidents. Use this as a map for your conversation: Identify what age or ages in your life you want to explore. For example, you may choose to want to gain insight into a formative accident you experienced at age 16. When you sit down with your grandparents, begin by asking, "What was your life like at 16?" (or whatever age in your own life you're examining); then follow up with, "What stands out to you as the most impactful experience in your life that year?" Keeping questions specific, rather than open-ended, can also be a useful tool for facilitating a more productive conversation—questions like, "Where did you live?" "Who did you live with?" "Did you experience any illnesses?" "What job did you have?" "What was your favorite book?" "Who was your best friend?" If you don't know them already, ask about the names of parents, siblings, and extended family. *Record their answers.* Yes, you can take notes as they talk, but wouldn't a video be a wonderful keepsake to have? Go year by year, should you want to explore larger portions of your life.

Give your grandparents space to share what they want. If you get a no, respect their decision without insisting. Communicate with respect and without judgment, as you would like others to relate to you. This is a crucial key for the family dynamic's well-being. Once you've spoken with your grandparents, review their answers and compare them to your own inventory. Look for repeated dates, experiences, etc. Look for any patterns. Trust yourself and relax into it. We are wired as humans to recognize patterns, even if it seems unlikely.

I hope this exercise will help you identify patterns in your own family and gain new insights about the ways in which you may be identified or entangled with family members—empowering you to disrupt old patterns. When we can see ourselves in the bigger picture, we can understand our fate in the context of the family system, which grounds us more firmly in our place in that system—better equipping us to chart our own destinies.

CHAPTER 3

The Only Right Parents

You Don't Have to Love Your Parents

Nine times out of ten, no matter what issue drives clients to reach out to me—a stalled career, a messy dating life, relationship woes, money trouble—we always, and I mean *always*, end up talking about their parents. Okay, yes, it is called *Family Constellations* for a reason. And, of course, many people come to me explicitly because of a difficult relationship with a parent or parents. In that way, Family Constellations may seem pretty similar to conventional therapy. If you've seen a therapist, after all, what was one of the first things they wanted to know about? I'm going to guess your childhood. There's an infamous saying about parents fucking you up. On that point, I'm willing to bet that 9 out of 10 therapists agree, regardless of what type of therapy they practice.

In my work, I've seen time and again how profoundly our relationship with our parents can affect our self-worth, our ability to form healthy relationships, our professional success, and our financial solvency, among other life dynamics. But when it comes to how to restore peace to those relationships, how to reconcile ourselves to a difficult parent dynamic, how to heal from the wounds we may have sustained in childhood and now carry in adulthood, well, that's where the initial similarity between conventional therapy and Family Constellations ends.

In my experience, conventional therapy too often focuses on who or what in our past is to blame for our current struggles. We are taught to rifle through the storehouse of our memories to uncover *who did what to us*, to identify ourselves as victims. In particular, we are encouraged to judge our parents: to catalog what was lacking in our childhood, to inventory our parents' shortcomings, the injuries we sustained from their abysmal parenting.

Of course, many of us do have parents who failed to meet our needs. We may have had a parent who was cold and unreceptive to our emotions, a parent who treated our feelings as an inconvenience, a parent who treated us as a surrogate for a partner, a parent whose expectations we could never meet, a parent who denied our identity, a parent who blurred boundaries (or never set them), a "rageaholic," an alcoholic, a parent who died early, or an otherwise absent parent. Even worse, too many of us have parents who were emotionally and/or physically abusive. Of course, our biological mother and father and the people who raised us—who parented us—are not always one and the same; we may have biological parents we never met (please note, in Family Constellations, all that follows applies to both, as you'll come to understand). These are facts. But too often, in therapy or just in life, we develop a narrative around these facts, a subjective story about what those facts mean about us.

We revisit this narrative often, as a way to assign responsibility to our parents for our current unhappiness, creating a kind of script—in which our role is victim—by which we live and limit our lives, abdicating agency. Our parents, not us, become responsible for our current choices, behaviors, and struggles. Even if you've never set foot in a therapist's office, you likely have a script of your own regarding your parents. Take a minute and check in with yourself. Grab a notebook or open a notes app on your phone. Close your eyes and visualize your parents. Send your awareness through your body. How does it feel? Tense? Tight? Relaxed? Now, with honesty, ask yourself (and note your answers), *Do I resent one or both of my parents? Why? What do I blame them for? How do I sit in judgment of that; what do I believe they should have done differently?* Writing down your answers to these questions is a way of gaining both clarity on how you feel and distance from it. When we "get out of our head," we create literal perspective as we commit our thoughts to paper and are able to view them separated from our interiority.

Now, make two lists: one titled "facts" and the other titled "narrative." Reread what you've written and see if you can tease apart the facts (what happened) from the narrative (what you believe those facts mean). For example, maybe your mother worked long hours and was often absent or unavailable in daily life or for school events, extracurriculars, or pivotal moments. Those are facts. How you feel about them, and yourself, is the narrative: "My mother prioritized her career above me." "My mother loved working more than she loved me." "It's my mother's fault I never learned how to make close relationships with women." "It's my mother's fault I'm a workaholic." "My mother didn't care enough about me to be there when I needed her." "My mother didn't—doesn't—love me enough." "I am not worthy of my mother's love." "I am fundamentally unworthy."

Do you see how damaging such a narrative would be? How it would turn into a script in which your role is to never be good enough in life and love and in which your own choices are now viewed as a natural consequence of your mother's actions (rather than your own values)? In our hypothetical case, it is true that the mother worked long hours. And it is true that the mother missed events of importance in the child's life. But the narrative itself—"My mother loved working more than she loved me"—is not provable; it is not a fact. If it were, the mother or other members of the household, such as siblings, would share an identical narrative. But of course they don't; they never do. Perhaps the mother's narrative sounds more like "I sacrificed to give my child the life I never had" or "My hard work modeled self-reliance and independence to my child after my divorce."

Not only is living by such a script incredibly disempowering (we are literally relinquishing our power over our own lives when we do this), but it is also a disavowal of life itself: When we live in the past, we reject the present. Even as we believe we are working to move forward, we are trapped in the dead zone of the past—a place without possibility for change or growth. Take a long, hard look at your narratives again: Where have you relinquished agency in your own life in favor of assigning blame to your parents? Where has your life grown stagnant while you've expended your time and energy resenting what your parents did or didn't do, what they could or couldn't give you, how they should have loved you differently or better?

When I met my client Jane, she was quarantining with her mother. Jane was in her late twenties and hadn't lived at home since she'd left for college. But Jane was a waitress, and when COVID-19 hit, she was furloughed. Rather than continue to pay rent in an expensive and tiny NYC apartment that she couldn't leave, she retreated back to her childhood home in New Jersey where she could live rent-free. On our first Zoom meeting, Jane spent the entire session talking about how much she couldn't stand her mom. She described how her mom had never loved her, had never truly seen her. She felt her sister had always received all of her mother's attention and that she had been treated like the ugly duckling. She had a long list of grievances that she relished enumerating in detail every time we spoke. Living with her mom had her in a state of constant fury; every little thing her mom did she took personally. She described her mom as passive-aggressive and calculating for not pouring her a cup of coffee. It was very interesting to me that despite how much Jane seemed to detest her mother, she had chosen to go back to her, especially at an unprecedented time of global insecurity and instability. "I had no choice, Marine," she insisted.

Jane's father had died four years earlier. She did not idealize him, however. In fact, quite the opposite: She viewed him as her mother's partner in crime, someone who was always disappointed in her and didn't believe in her. In fact, Jane was annoyed that her mother was still mourning her husband ("She acts like they had this perfect marriage, but they argued constantly," she griped). Her biggest complaint about her mom? "She's living in the past!" Jane was suffering from panic attacks and anxiety. She hated waitressing but had no clue about what she might want to do instead. She didn't seem to believe there was anything else she could do. She felt resentful of and insecure around her friends from college, all of whom were pursuing careers. She didn't believe in herself or know who she was. Sound familiar?

In retreating back to her mother's house, Jane was retreating to safety—the safety of her narrative. COVID-19 was the perfect alibi. Jane didn't have to take responsibility for anything anymore. To her thinking, she had no choice. Working with Jane was a little like playing whack-a-mole; every time we reached a resolution, a newly remembered grievance would pop up that she would cite as a reason it really was her parents' fault that x, y, or z wasn't playing out in her life the way she'd hoped.

Over the course of our sessions, Jane was able to start getting out of her head. Blame is a kind of fixated thinking. As she got out of her head, she was able to reconnect with her body. Jane was shut down. She didn't want to feel her emotions, which was part of why she'd been having the panic attacks. They were like her body's SOS system. Jane's parents had been emotionally shut down, and she had internalized the idea that feelings weren't safe. As Jane grew more comfortable feeling her feelings, she was increasingly able to take ownership of them, especially how much she did love her parents—and how afraid of that love she was. She was able to tap into that love, her own agency, and relinquish the narrative she'd been grasping so desperately. By reengaging and reconnecting with her emotions, she was finally able to see the truth: She just wanted to be loved and seen, and when she started seeing and loving herself, things became much easier. She was no longer chasing after her parents; instead, she was giving herself what she needed and so what her inner child needed. Finally aligned with her authentic needs, Jane was accepted to a master's program to become an occupational therapist—and she moved out of her mom's home on good terms.

When we engage in blaming and judging our parents, we are not only rejecting the present, we are also rejecting them. What we reject, we repeat. What we reject, we exclude. This is why in Family Constellations we don't play the blame game (as they say in the States, "Play stupid games, win stupid prizes"). When we exclude a parent or parents from our Family System, we create disorder in the system, imbalance. Remember, the Family System will always seek to restore its balance and integrity, primarily through entanglement.

Our well-being depends on giving our parents their rightful place in our family system. We must restore their belonging, however resistant we are to such an idea or how unpleasant it may feel initially. Because reconciliation doesn't come—*cannot* come—through identifying how our parents fucked us up and leaving it at that, even if we have a goal of eventually forgiving them. Acceptance, not forgiveness, is the key to changing the dynamic with our parents.

This doesn't mean we don't assign our parents responsibility for their actions, of course not. They are responsible for what they did. We don't excuse and we don't forgive. In Family Constellations we always emphasize an individual's responsibility for his or her actions; once you are an adult, you are always solely accountable for your choices and your actions. So it bears repeating, your parents are solely responsible for their actions. But this also means *you are not in charge of what is their responsibility.*

Maybe this seems obvious. But in a sense, when you fixate on your parents' mistakes or shortcomings and you wish for retribution—or even forgiveness—you are attempting to control the outcomes of their choices, to deliver their fate, something that is not in your power. You cannot take on responsibility for another's actions; you have to leave them to their fate (remember, this is what we mean when we talk about respecting someone else's fate). Don't waste your own energy and resources and risk or perpetuate entanglement by inserting yourself in their fate.

When I first met my client Jonathan, he had just sold his first start-up for a tidy sum and raised a substantial amount of capital for his next project. He was in his early thirties, healthy, and now wealthy. He should have been reveling in his hard-earned success, but instead he was struggling with intense anxiety. Every night he had dreams that he'd been sent to prison, without a trial, and with a sentence of unknown length. About a decade earlier, I was surprised to learn, Jonathan had been in prison. In his early twenties, he had robbed a convenience store. While he was in prison, his sister gave him a copy of Don Miguel Ruiz's *The Four Agreements*, a spiritual code of conduct that set him on a path of personal growth and spiritual development. Jonathan became a model prisoner: He began studying coding, took accountability for his actions, and helped other prisoners prep for their appeals and court dates. After he was released early for good behavior, he applied and was admitted to a prestigious computer science program. By the time I met Jonathan, he was fully "reformed." Listening to him describe his past was like listening to someone describe a character in a novel. But despite his years of clean living, he was haunted by a fear that somehow he would end up in a dark place again, almost as if he were not in control of his own life. He couldn't enjoy his success, and though he felt ready to start a family, he had little luck with dating.

After Jonathan brought me up to speed on his adult life, we started his constellation. This was a "blind" constellation: Prior to the constellation, based on our conversations and the issues Jonathan told me he wanted to work on, I had made a list of who would be included. I knew who each set of "footsteps" represented, but Jonathan did not. Jonathan laid them out, and then we went set by set as Jonathan described how he felt in relation to each pair. Once Jonathan was finished, I revealed who each set of footsteps represented, and we revisited what he had said about each. When we were done talking about his constellation and the insights we drew from it, I realized with some embarrassment that we were missing a pair of footsteps and I hadn't noticed. Far in the corner of the desk where we had laid out the constellation was the last pair, the ones that represented Jonathan's father. Even I, the therapist, had completely forgotten them. When I asked Jonathan what he was feeling, he answered, "Nothing . . . I don't feel anything." I gently revealed to Jonathan that the footsteps represented his father. "Huh," Jonathan responded. It quickly became clear that he literally had no idea where his father was. "I don't know, and I don't care," he said. "I haven't seen him since I was a little kid, and I literally never even think about him anymore." Jonathan then explained to me that when he was five years old, his dad went to prison for robbing a bank. His mother had divorced his father while he was in prison; they never visited him, and his mother had assiduously avoided even talking about him after that. When she did mention him, it was as a cautionary tale ("Don't become like your father") or as a contrast to Jonathan's own behavior ("You're so much smarter/better/kinder than your father"). Once she remarried, any mention at all of Jonathan's father became verboten.

"I know, it's kind of a cliché: My dad went to prison, I grew up without a dad, then I went to prison." Jonathan shrugged. "I've kind of hammered that to death in therapy already." In Jonathan's view, he had worked to forgive his father and move on, claiming that *he didn't think about him anymore.* He assumed the prison dreams were just stress-induced. But Jonathan had never stopped blaming his father. He had never readmitted him into the fold of his family system, had never truly accepted him *as his father.* He lived in an ongoing state of rejection, especially of his own life and the possibility of becoming a father himself. Jonathan was clearly entangled with his father, subconsciously loyal to the man who had been excluded, and taking up his fate in order to take his place, despite his protests to the contrary.

In the constellation, Jonathan was able to offer his father a return to his rightful place. He addressed his father, first with a simple declaration of acceptance: "Dad, I am your son; you are my father." Then he stepped away from blame and established a boundary: "You did the best you could; I'll take it from here." By respecting his father's right of belonging, Jonathan was able to sever the entanglement. He had no desire to seek out his father or develop a relationship with him, but by no longer denying his paternity, as it were, he was able to reconcile himself to life as it is, to life itself. The dreams stopped, as did his unspoken fear that he would be an unfit father.

I know, it feels good to blame our parents. There is a delicious quality to the righteous anger we experience when we can enumerate the ways that the people who were supposed to love us the most hurt us instead. And there is a perverse sense of safety, of comfort even, in the victim role, despite how it continually shunts us back to the source of discomfort and pain, because it is both familiar and also functions as a protective excuse. But you are an adult now and you do have power—you get to determine your relationships and your choices around them. The only person you can count on to change the dynamic with your parents, to disrupt the pattern, is you.

Yes, it's challenging when we have to deal with toxic people or dynamics. It's even more challenging and hurtful when those people are our mother or father. But to remain in a place of victimhood—to constantly cry out, "It's not fair, why me?!"—is to reject responsibility for your life and to disempower yourself. Complaining, blaming, and whining are toxic for our well-being. These defensive behaviors undermine our power. When we cut them out, we make the choice to grant ourselves a higher value and to stand up for our real self. Love is preceded by respect. When we respect ourselves, we will automatically bring love back.

We cannot change the past, even if it *wasn't* fair, but we can control our relationship to it. We can lay down our anger, pain, and disappointment. We can, as always, stop arguing with reality and acknowledge what is: Our parents are our parents. The only option is to let go of any expectations and take what they have to give, however limited it may be, exactly as it is. You don't have to love your parents, but you do have to accept them.

This is where the rubber hits the road when it comes to our parents, though. I'm warning you: This next part is a little tough. This is where my clients often balk. Because it would be nice—easy even, if a bit Pollyannaish—if I told you all we had to do to achieve reconciliation is let go of our expectations. But when it comes to our parents, acknowledging what is means not only accepting and agreeing to the reality that our parents are our parents, but also acknowledging that *our parents are the only right parents for us.*

Yikes. Never mind your regular-old parental disfunction, how can we ever say that harmful parents are the only right parents for us? And why do we need to? In the most basic sense, our parents are the only right parents for us because they are our only parents. Without them, we wouldn't be. Bert Hellinger wrote, "There are no other parents than these. Therefore they are the best parents, the only possible parents, and therefore also the only right parents."[1] Our existence depends on the reality of the two particular people who combined their genetic inheritance to create us. There is no other path to life except through those two particular people. Therefore, they are the only right people—what they were like is, for all intents and purposes, irrelevant. In this way, the mere fact of creating life makes them "the only right parents."

But why does it matter whether or not we acknowledge this? Let's pause for a minute. Close your eyes, allow yourself to relax, and bring your awareness to your heartbeat. With every beat of your heart, you are feeling the force of life that moves through you. This life came to you through your biological parents. Whether you knew them or not, life moved through them to you. Regardless of the quality of their parenting, they transmitted that life force in full; there is nothing they could take from it or add to it. And through this gift of life, your parents necessarily connect you to something greater and deeper than yourself—not only to the chain of ancestors who precede you but to the source of life itself, whatever that may be. When we can reach the place of acknowledging that *our parents are the only right parents for us,* we are in a state of complete and total submission to the force of life itself, and therefore in a full embrace of it.

In order to live a life that is truly vibrant, replete with vitality and fulfillment, we must receive as much of that life force as possible. As children of our parents, that's really our only job: to take whatever it is they have to offer, which is life itself. When we cut ourselves off from our parents, deny our parents, reject or exclude our parents, in our hearts or minds, we are diverting the flow of life away from ourselves. This doesn't mean you have to have a close relationship with your parents. Many of us don't know our biological parents: You may be adopted, or your parent may have used an egg or sperm donor. And, as we discussed, many of us have parents who were abusive or who are otherwise toxic people. Agreeing that *our parents are the only right parents for us* does not mean agreeing to abuse. The great Family Constellations facilitator Dr. Joy Manné writes that she helps clients who have suffered parental abuse meet this difficult task by having them state, "Now I take you as my [father/mother], and I agree to the price of what it cost you, and what it costs me."[2] I love this statement because it both reinforces the responsibility of the parent ("what it cost you" = the parent's fate) while also honoring the experience of the child ("what it costs me").

Acknowledging and accepting that your parents are the only right parents for you means opening yourself to receiving what they have to offer, fundamentally: life itself. Doing so is not mutually exclusive with having boundaries (e.g., choosing not to be in communication with toxic parents). Finding the right distance between ourselves and our parents, biological or otherwise, is one of the greatest gifts we can give ourselves. But we can't create those boundaries or experience true autonomy if our parents aren't there, figuratively speaking, to separate from. There is no right distance to measure; their absence in the family system instead creates a kind of gravity well, pulling us further into a dysfunctional dynamic rather than keeping us safe. Reincluding our parents in our family system means putting them in their right place—and when they're in their right place, we are free to leave them be. The systemic consciousness doesn't need to seek anyone to fill the holes they left behind.

AFFIRMATIONS

I am not in charge of your responsibility.

You are my only right parents.

Life flows through you to me.

Thank you for the gift of life.

EXERCISE: Take a Bow

---

*"We bow down before the life that has come to us,
just as it has come to us, with everything it entails,
and we take it as such into our hearts and our souls."*

— BERT HELLINGER, PEACE BEGINS IN THE SOUL

Although it's a simple movement, bowing can be a challenging act. It requires us to set aside our egos. When we bow, we make ourselves physically humble before another, whether that other is divine or human. It is an act of trust—in bowing, we literally make ourselves vulnerable, exposing our heads and necks, limiting our line of sight. Outside the West (where the handshake tends to rule supreme, at least prior to COVID-19), the bow is a standard greeting across many cultures, as well as an act of respect, reverence, and devotion. When actors bow at the end of a performance, they are signaling their gratitude to the audience, their gratitude for our act of witnessing their art; their creation; in a sense, their creative force—their life force. That feeling at the end of an incredible theater experience, when the actors make their way onstage and we lose ourselves in clapping as they take their bows, is exhilarating for us, as well. We can feel life itself coursing between us at that moment.

One way to practice receiving the life force your parents have to offer—to accept them as the only right parents—is to bow before them, to bow before life itself. Okay, not *literally* before them. But, if you are ready to try, you can use a photo to represent them or any object you associate either with your parents or with the idea of parenting and parenthood. I once had a client who used a muslin swaddle blanket to represent parenthood and another who used a coffee cup from a set that her parents drank from every weekend morning when she was growing up. If you are not ready to bow to an image of your parents or to an object emblematic of your parents or parenthood in general, you can bow to something that resonates with life, like a healthy houseplant.

Find a quiet space where you have room to set out a yoga mat, towel, or blanket that will be comfortable for kneeling. Set your object in front of you, elevated on a small table or a stack of books (get as creative as you need to here). Then, kneel before it and lower your upper body to the floor (think Child's Pose in yoga). As you bow, try reciting any of the above affirmations. Hold the bow for at least 10 seconds and bring your awareness to your body. Feel your own life force—your heartbeat, your breath—as you rest supported in the flow of life.

Receiving and Taking

In accepting your parents as the only right parents, you are necessarily accepting that your mother and your father, *in their separate roles*, are your only right mother and father. You can't accept one and not the other; it simply doesn't work that way. Not only does your existence require their genetic union, but you must also acknowledge that your parents already chose one another—their fates are, in a sense, inextricably bound. This remains true regardless of how well they knew each other (pregnancy doesn't discriminate between a one-night stand and a long-term relationship) or whether they knew each other at all (even in the case of sperm donation, for example, there is the obvious choice the mother makes in picking the donor, but there is also the choice the donor makes to create life with the anonymous recipient).

As we touched on, our biological mother and father and the people who raised us—who parented us—are not always one and the same. But, as human beings, we all arrive earthside through the merging of an ovum and sperm, through the coming together of a female life force on one hand and a male life force on the other. Through that inheritance, each of us carries an admixture of feminine and masculine energies, regardless of our gender identity.

Each of those energies, each legacy, enriches your life; when you reject one, not only that part of yourself but also those associated parts of your life—success, creativity, or health, among other aspects—are stifled. In their purest form, these energies are the essence of receiving (the feminine) and taking (the masculine). Again, these energies are not correlated to our gender expression; every person contains both, to different degrees, regardless of whether they identify as male, female, or nonbinary. Think of the ability to receive as the ability to be *open*: to be open to others, to ideas, to intuition, to be receptive and perceptive. Think of the ability to take as the ability to take action: to be decisive, to be purposeful, to be oriented toward a goal, to be analytical in our assessments. The feminine and the masculine are complementary energies. For each of us, they interlock in unique ways that shape who we are, what we value, how we understand ourselves, and how we approach the world. When one or the other is rejected, we suffer for it; we all need both in order to thrive. Being able to receive these energies and embrace them in every way that they manifest in our lives begins with accepting their source: the first woman and the first man in our lives, our biological parents.

In my experience, most people do have a more difficult relationship with one parent than the other. Very often, that parent is their mother. Let's be honest: We tend to hold our mothers to a standard we rarely set for anyone else in our lives. And we live in a culture that already expects so much more of mothers than fathers, setting a bar for women that almost none can meet—because it isn't a bar at all, but a moving target designed to always be just out of reach. (Meanwhile, the bar for fathers is on the floor.)

Never mind that that moving target itself operates in a minefield of sexism and gender-based inequities. So please, when I say that in examining your current issues and relationships, the first and most important person to consider is the mother, the second most important person is the mother, and the third most important person is the mother, know that while I *am* being a bit cheeky, I'm in no way suggesting that our mothers are somehow the source of everything woe begotten in our lives. Instead, I'm underscoring a simple reality: Women give birth.

Look, it is through our mothers, quite literally, that we enter this world. For nine months she carries us within her (and indeed, when a woman is pregnant, she contains within her the life force of three generations: her own, that of her unborn child, and that of the generation following, which is already an aspect of her baby). In giving birth, she risks her life for our own (even now, when science and medicine have reduced this risk, it is still deeply embedded in our shared human psyche). Women carry the greater weight in ensuring the survival of the species.

Our mother is the first woman in our life, and our life depends on her. Our relationship with her—one of ultimate vulnerability—is our first experience of being in relationship, however brief. All our future relationships (platonic or romantic) are a link in a chain that begins there, in our mother's arms. The mother is the primary source of caring, of comfort, of nurturance. She creates and sustains life. For all of these reasons and more, the mother is the archetype of the feminine.

When we reject our mother, we're essentially rejecting all that is archetypally feminine. As a result, we may hold ourselves at a remove from those things we associate subconsciously with mothering: security, safety, comfort, care. We may not care for ourselves; we may not care for or connect with our bodies, damaging our health as a result or alienating ourselves from our sensuality and sexuality. We may struggle with intimacy, physical or emotional. We may not care for our homes and our environment, letting them lapse into states of disarray or worse. We may simply not feel at home in the world. We may struggle with money, a major source of security. We may struggle to hear the trusted voice of our intuition speaking to us. Our creativity, such as our ability to write, create art, make music, and problem solve, may be blocked, and our ability to connect to the creative—to be moved to tears by a piece of music, say, or to have our perspective changed by a novel, a film, or a painting—may be deadened. Simply put, in order to embrace the feminine, we must embrace our mother.

Whether or not you feel you have any overt issues with your mother, ask yourself how you would describe her. Do you feel connected or disconnected to her? What was she like in your childhood? What are the first words that come to mind when you think of her? Write out your answer: You can simply write a list of adjectives as they come to you or, if it comes more naturally, freewrite your response as you would a journal entry. Don't belabor it either way—the idea is to connect with your immediate associations.

Where might you struggle with the feminine in your life? For example, are you able to receive help when it's offered? Do you feel present in your body, attuned to your own sensuality? Do you feel confident in your ability to take care of yourself? If you identify as a woman, are you able to support and hold up other women in your life, especially in arenas that you might perceive as having limited opportunities, such as work? If you identify as a man, have you had meaningful platonic relationships with women outside of your family, such as with a teacher or mentor? Are you able to connect with your creativity, either through your ability to appreciate the work of others or through your own creative pursuits? Again, write out your answer and try not to overthink it, though I grant that this question is a bit less concrete.

Now read over what you've written. Do you see any connections between the language you used to describe your mother and your attitudes and experience of the feminine?

For my client Vivienne, a rigidly controlled life was the dark shadow of her shame and anger surrounding her mother. Vivienne came to me at an emotionally fraught moment in her life: Her mother was seriously ill with cancer and had moved in with Vivienne and her children. Vivienne was now her mother's caretaker. Although she did not exactly resent this obligation, it did reopen painful wounds: Throughout Vivienne's childhood, her mother had been largely absent, more a glittery apparition than any kind of remotely consistent presence.

Vivienne had been conceived at Woodstock, the product of a muddy fling between two passionate hippies who never saw each other again. Vivienne had no idea who her father was, and her mother seemed completely uninterested in the subject. When I mentioned how remarkable the story of her conception was—after all, Woodstock is a historic event of major cultural significance—Vivienne seemed surprised. "It just seems like it would have been really loud, wet, and dirty," she said with a shrug. The presence of legends like Jimi Hendrix and Janis Joplin at the moment of her conception elicited a giant *meh*.

After she was born, Vivienne was raised by her maternal grandmother, while her mother pursued her dreams of being an actress. Vivienne described her mother as unconventional, wild, free, remarkably beautiful, highly desired, and sexually open in a way that was socially unacceptable at the time ("She slept around, to put it mildly," Vivienne said dryly). Though all of those qualities could be interpreted as admirable, Vivienne's expression as she listed them suggested a terrible stench had permeated the room. As an actress, her mother had gone on to perform in sexually explicit "art films." "I think they were probably just pornography," Vivienne said. "I was ashamed and embarrassed of her."

When Vivienne was a teenager, her mother returned home for good. Vivienne found her intrusion into her and her grandmother's life deeply uncomfortable. "She didn't know who I was or the first thing about me as a person. She behaved like I was still two or three—the last time she'd spent more than a day with me—instead of sixteen. And she was still insanely beautiful—much prettier than me—and uninterested in concealing her sexuality, right as I was mired in the awkwardness of my own changing body and growing awareness of sex." Vivienne found her mother to be impossibly immature; she would often lose her keys, borrow money from Vivienne, and request rides into town. "It was like I was the adult, and she was the child." I asked Vivienne if she thought her mother loved her. "Yes," Vivienne said unhesitatingly, "but she was selfish. She never grew up or accepted responsibility for anything."

Vivienne herself was a striking woman and presented in a highly "feminine" manner: I never saw her without her hair blown out, her makeup impeccable, her manicure glossy. She had an elegant style, but it was all highly controlled. Vivienne radiated a kind of inflexibility—she was strict about exercise and what she ate, but, by her own admission, completely out of tune with her own physical pleasure. She was divorced and hadn't had sex in several years. "Sex has never been my strong suit," she said ruefully. Beyond maintaining her appearance, Vivienne did not engage in any kind of self-care. "I don't have time for that," she explained. "I'm a single mother, and I have my kids to take care of, and now my mother."

Vivienne wanted partnership and a fulfilling sex life but found dating almost impossible. She struggled to be open to men, never making it past three or four dates before her walls would go up as things started to get more personal. And she was not receptive to anyone who didn't conform to her idea of what successful adult life should look like—the "right" kind of education, the "right" kind of job. Vivienne's whole life struck me as an act of denial: She denied herself love, comfort, relaxation, spontaneity, companionship, just as she denied her mother. In taking her mother into her home, she was in many ways reenacting her mother's "intrusion" into her life 30 years earlier. In caring for her mother through her illness, she was forced yet again to contend with her mother's physicality, just as she had in adolescence. And now she was racked with guilt that she was still so angry with this person who had given her life, even as her mother approached the end of her own life.

Vivienne's resolution was powerful and beautiful to witness. In our first blind constellation, Vivienne set her mother's footsteps in front of her own. "How do you feel?" I asked. "Sad and confused," Vivienne said. "I want to go to them, but I'm afraid." Vivienne and her mother were not in their right places. Vivienne had been denying her mother her rightful place in the constellation— there was a gap behind her where her mother should have been. She felt a sensation that she had no one immediately to fall back on. When Vivienne returned her mother's footsteps to their place of belonging behind her, she visibly relaxed. "I'm sorry I judged you, Mom," she said. "I accept how you lived your life, and I take what you have to offer." Vivienne described feeling a new strength at her back. In our next session, Vivienne worked on setting clear boundaries with her mother, boundaries that had been violated in childhood when Vivienne had been privy to information about her mother's sex life. "Mom, I leave you to your business; it is none of mine," she said. "I am your daughter, not your mother. You are the mother."

Over our next sessions, she found that as her mother was no longer "in front of her," she was better able to see her own children, who were approaching adolescence themselves. As she let go of her shame centered on her mother's sexuality, she began to feel more empowered to explore her own. At age 46, she bought her first vibrator. She felt empowered by her femininity and sexuality, rather than burdened by its obligations. She spent less time grooming herself to "perfection" and more time listening to her body; she dropped the cardio classes and took up swimming, feeling supported and unencumbered in the water, a sort of return to the womb. She felt tenderness in caring for her mother, tending the gift of life her mother had once transmitted to her. In accepting her mother, Vivienne was able to embrace the feminine, and in embracing the feminine, Vivienne was finally receptive to the strength and power that were part of her mother's legacy.

Our relationships with our fathers are no less important than the ones we have with our mothers, but they often involve more distance, both physical and emotional, which can make them seem secondary. The bonds with our mothers start in utero, whereas a father's bond with his child has a more abstract quality until the birth itself. And, historically, men have severed that bond—discarding their responsibility to it—more easily and with more frequency. The creation of another life has fewer concrete consequences for men: They don't have to carry the child; they don't have to give birth; they don't have to recover from birth; they don't have to nurse. You'd *think* with so few initial demands on them, the bar for what fathers are supposed to do should be quite high, but you'd be wrong. The bar for fathers is so much lower than it is for mothers—change a diaper and a father is practically anointed a superhero. Instead, we learn, culturally, that it is our mother whom we should hold to a rigorous standard, leading us to so often feel she has failed to meet it. With our fathers, interestingly, we often feel it is *they* who are holding *us* to a standard we can't meet.

This feeling is enforced by a culture that denigrates the feminine and perverts the masculine. Every person contains both feminine and masculine energies. I know I've said as much several times already, but it bears repeating. Feminine energy qualities such as expressiveness, emotion, intuition, and receptiveness are profoundly necessary qualities for living well and deeply, especially in relationship with other people—but our culture often treats these as weak and teaches boys and men that they are to be feared and avoided. Meanwhile, necessary and equally beautiful masculine energy qualities such as structure, logic, and reason are exploited in service to ego and power. They become overemphasized and have no counterbalance. Thus the father can be a figure who is unfeeling and rigid, who wields dominance and requires submission. In Judeo-Christian culture, the archetypal Father is the authority to whom we answer.

When we set aside the ways in which our culture has twisted masculine energy, we can better see how profoundly we need those qualities, how they make a functioning and meaningful life possible. As with our mothers and the feminine, accepting the masculine in our life begins with accepting the first man in our life—our biological father—regardless of how he expressed that masculinity, regardless of how present he was, and regardless of the other men who may have stepped up to father us in his absence. The father is the shelter, the protector, the guide, the explorer. He makes and guards the space in which the mother can focus on nurturing; he sets out into the world to bring back that which makes ongoing care possible.

When we reject our father, we're essentially rejecting all that is archetypally masculine. As a result, we may hold ourselves at a remove from those things we associate subconsciously with the father: the ability to protect ourselves and others, authority *over our own lives*, the building of skills, loyalty, adventure. We may struggle with honoring our commitments; we may have difficulty holding on to friendships and relationships; we may fear the unknown and lack the spirit to go outside our comfort zone, never realizing our full abilities; we may rebuff reasoned decision-making and struggle with impulsiveness; our lives may feel desultory and haphazard, as if they are happening to us rather than through our will.

Whether or not you feel you have any overt issues with your father, ask yourself how you would describe him. Do you feel connected or disconnected to him? What was he like in your childhood? What are the first words that come to mind when you think of him? Write out your answer: You can simply write a list of adjectives as they come to you or, if it comes more naturally, freewrite your response as you would a journal entry. Don't belabor it either way—the idea is to connect with your immediate associations.

Where might you struggle with the masculine in your life? For example, are you able to ask for help when you need to? (Note that asking is different from receiving.) Do you feel confident in your ability to set boundaries and guard your well-being? Do you set goals and see them through, or do you falter when making decisions and lack the will to initiate change? If you identify as a man, do you have meaningful platonic relationships with men in which you feel comfortable talking about your life? If you identify as a woman, do you have close relationships with men (not including fathers or romantic partners) whom you are not seeking to please?

Are you able to connect with the spirit of adventure, be that through seeking out new ideas, trying unfamiliar foods, engaging in challenging activities? Do you challenge yourself in general? Again, write out your answers and try not to overthink them.

Now read over what you've written. Do you see any connections between the language you used to describe your father and your attitudes and experience of the masculine?

For Pierre, his father was not absent, but his mother was the sun around which he revolved. Pierre was the youngest of three kids. He had two older sisters and was not only the baby but also the only boy. As a result, his mother doted on him, and their relationship was highly enmeshed. Pierre seemed to completely disavow any importance his father played in his life. "He worked all the time," he said. He described his father as boring, remote, and shut down. "When he came home from work, he watched TV. But not even, like, shows, just cable news," he said, rolling his eyes. On weekends, rather than spend time with his kids, Pierre's father played tennis with his brother, Pierre's uncle. "We don't have anything to say to each other," Pierre told me about their present-day relationship.

Pierre described his mother as effervescent, the life of the party, everyone's best friend, and the perfect homemaker—an incredible cook, super crafty, with an eye for beauty. "I don't even know what my mom saw in my dad," he told me. "They are complete opposites. My mom was so lively and fun; she always made time to play with us; she had an incredible imagination; she invented the best games." The ways in which Pierre described his mom struck me as strangely arrested; it was as if he were still a child reciting why "Mommy is the best." There was no mention of any qualities that an *adult* child might find worthy of mentioning about his parent.

Pierre had come to me because his marriage was falling apart. His wife wanted to divorce, and he was heartbroken. He expressed surprise that divorce was happening to him (his words), given that his own parents had been married for almost 40 years. He seemed to think that only people from "broken homes" got divorced.

One thing I want to note here is that, interestingly, idealization is also a form of rejection. When we idealize a parent, we refuse them the reality of who they are as complex people with all that comes with that, good and bad. When we reject the less-than-ideal aspects of a person by insisting that there are none (refusing to see them), we are not seeing the person in front of us in the fullness of their humanity.

Pierre idealized his mom as he simultaneously rejected his father. His father wasn't "good enough" for his perfect mother. And now, Pierre's wife wasn't good enough for him; she had told him in no uncertain terms that she felt he constantly belittled and undermined her. Pierre acknowledged that he sometimes "suggested" different ways she should do things—the way his mother had done them. But no matter what Pierre's wife did or didn't do, it wouldn't have mattered; she couldn't have met his expectations, because they were based on his imaginary construction of his larger-than-life mother. Pierre reported that his wife complained that he constantly made her promises he didn't keep, especially regarding seeing a marriage counselor, and that she was unhappy with his unwillingness to ever try anything new. She felt Pierre was controlling and that their life and marriage had become stifling and stale.

Meanwhile, Pierre grappled with an array of insecurities: The neighborhood he and his wife lived in was not the safest, and he felt ashamed they couldn't afford to move; Pierre had been passed up for a promotion at work because, as his boss said, he lacked initiative. He worried about providing for future children and felt that his sisters looked down on him. The only woman Pierre seemed to have a positive relationship with was his mother. Once a week, he still drove 60 miles there and back for dinner at his parents' home. "I only go because of my mom," he said. I asked if his dad joined the dinners. "Yes, but it's awkward," he reported. "Last time I was there, he asked if I want to come up and play tennis sometime. I hate when he asks because I always have to come up with an excuse." It turned out Pierre's father had been inviting him to join him for a match every week for years and that Pierre had, indeed, played tennis with his father when he was a kid. "It was boring, though," he said. "I hate tennis."

When we did Pierre's first constellation, he resisted what it revealed to him: that his real issue in his marriage was not his wife, their inability to communicate, or even her relationship with his mom, who, Pierre reported, adored his wife—it was his idealization of his mother and his resulting disconnect from his father. Pierre was deeply alienated from the masculine in his life, and he was paralyzed as a result. It made sense that Pierre described his mother as though he were still a child: Adulthood and its attendant demands overwhelmed him. He was also unavailable to his wife; his constellation revealed that he already occupied the position of his mother's partner, usurping his father's place in the meantime.

As Pierre stepped out of position and into his right spot, making room for his father to take his place, he expressed his regret: "Dad, I'm sorry there was never room for you between me and Mom." Though he did not blame his mother, he could see that she had created an unhealthy dynamic. He accepted that she had likely been caught up in a lingering family dynamic of her own, and established a boundary for himself: "Mom, I love you, but I am your son, not your partner." In the days following the constellation, Pierre began to feel a lightening in his body. He felt more energetic, less tired. He researched an accreditation course that would help him level up in his career and signed up for night classes. He asked his wife to go to marriage counseling. And he began occasionally playing tennis with his dad. Each time he and his dad played, Pierre felt more and more at peace. "We don't really talk much, but just being on the court together, there's a kind of rhythm we connect in." I couldn't help but think of the child development concept of the "serve and return," which describes a child/caregiver dynamic much like a game of tennis. In the serve-and-return dynamic, an infant "serves" by attempting interaction—making eye contact, babbling, gesturing—and a caregiver "returns" the serve by mirroring the action: responding to the babble, imitating the gesture, smiling back. The serve and return teaches us how to connect. In making room for his father, Pierre was making room for the masculine, making room for himself, room to grow and stop resisting authority over his own life. In stepping back from the idealized version of his mother, Pierre made even more room for the authentic feminine within himself and in others, particularly his wife.

The reasons we might reject our parents are complex. With our mother, we can always trace it back to a break in our bond; we may have experienced a literal separation from our mother in early childhood (e.g., she may have been hospitalized, she may have had to leave the country to attend to family issues of her own, etc.) that interrupted our "reaching-out movement" (in Family Constellations we call this "the interrupted movement"). In other words, you reached for your mother—you needed her—and she wasn't there. Such an interrupted movement teaches us that we can't rely on another person to meet our needs, and so we often defensively stop reaching altogether. More likely, you experienced an emotional break in a bond: Maybe you felt that your mother was self-absorbed, unavailable to you, uninterested in you, or didn't see you for who you were. You may have had to occupy the role of a partner rather than that of a child, breaking the right and real bond.

Our rejection of our fathers often stems from a sense that we have of being rejected, of a distance we did not choose. As infants, we share a kind of intimacy with our mothers that we don't with our fathers, which can be difficult for a new father to find space for himself in. Both physical and emotional distance are prevalent in dynamics with fathers—fathers who leave, fathers who were never in the picture, fathers who are workaholics, fathers who cannot express their love and hold themselves at a distance despite the love they feel. Many of us experienced authoritarian or dominant fathers who treated the family and the home as extensions of their will. Many of us, in relation to our fathers, feel that we will never be "good enough."

Whatever the reason your parent did not love you as you needed or wanted (and we will explore all of these dynamics and their legacies in more detail when we delve into extended family dynamics and relationships in the following chapters), it likely felt personal to you. How could it not? But the truth is, it likely had nothing to do with you (which may sting even more). We tend to see our parents as capital-P PARENTS—the role subsumes the entirety of their identity for us, their children. But it is unlikely that this is how they see themselves, because, of course, our parents had their own lives long before we came along. Our mothers and fathers had, and have, their own hopes and aspirations, their own struggles, their own family systems, their own inherited as well as personal traumas. When we experience a lack of love from a parent, the love may not have been available to give. Despite his or her love for you, their attention and focus may have been diverted by those traumas. It doesn't matter what it was or whether or not you know about it; you just need to know that the source of the behavior *lay within them*, not you. They did what they could with the tools they had.

In my own relationship with my mother, I spent many unhappy years demanding and insisting (not overtly, but through the way I related to her) that because she was the adult and my mother, she had to understand my way of thinking, take care of me as I wanted, and love me as I expected. To me, my mother was perfect, a kind of superwoman—she was incredibly intelligent, a successful lawyer, beautiful, kind, and life seemed to come easy for her. Honestly, I envied her. Even as I raised her up on a pedestal, I created resentment, because I felt that my life was unfairly difficult in comparison: I was sensitive and vulnerable, where my mother was blithe and untroubled, I believed, and thus I felt she owed me.

My mother was my hero, but she was also my unwitting antagonist. I saw myself as the victim of her choices. I was deeply angry about my experience in England, a trip my parents had arranged, and I was angry about their divorce, as I felt I had paid the bigger price, a price I never agreed to: my father's abandonment of me. Not only did my mother not struggle as I did, I believed, but she had added ongoing pain to my load. (She struggled, of course, but selfishly enough, I thought only of me.)

Over time, through therapeutic practices like and including Family Constellations, I came to understand that she was a woman with multiple facets that produced the particular kind of mother she was. As I came to understand that my mom was not only not perfect but also not capable of perfection, I began to allow her to make mistakes. Understanding that my mom was flawed was immensely liberating, because I stopped holding *myself* to a standard I could never meet. I also stopped seeing myself as being in competition with her—even though I wouldn't have described it that way at the time, that's what comparison is, a type of competition. When I stopped competing with her, I became less self-centered and more interested in her perspective. We began having long conversations about her life and experience. Our relationship began to feel intentional rather than inevitable. I chose her. Or rather, I chose to accept her as she is. Though I would always have described my relationship with my mother as close, true closeness came when I stopped being a "mommy's girl." My obsessive love for her transformed into a more authentic or enlightened love, in which I welcomed her in my heart in the fullness of her humanity, seeing her for who she is and accepting what she has to give, exactly as it is.

Parenting well is an incredibly difficult task, and some of us arrive there better equipped than others. It's inevitable that even "good" parents will make mistakes and hurt their children, though they don't intend to do so. The problem isn't really what our parents did to us but the harm we do to ourselves by holding on to it. When we make a demand about how our mothers or fathers should be or what they should have done for us, we cannot take what they do have to offer, however limited it may be. Accepting that your mother or father is the only right one for you means accepting what they have to give, exactly as it is.

AFFIRMATIONS

I embrace the feminine within me;

I embrace the masculine within me.

Mom/Dad, you are the only right mother/father for me.

Mom/Dad, you do not have to prove your love for me.

Mom/Dad, I take your love just as you give it.

EXERCISE: Practicing the Movement

"Such interruptions are accompanied by strong feelings of hurt, rejection, despair, hate, resignation, and grief. These feelings overlay the primal love, but they're just the reverse side of love. When young children can't reach the person they love, they have a strong tendency to feel rejected, as if there were something wrong with them, and they stop practicing the movement."

— BERT HELLINGER, LOVE'S HIDDEN SYMMETRY

The interrupted movement—a break in a bond—is one of the deepest wounds a child can sustain. Such interruptions often occur when we are too young to remember them, however, or they may not seem traumatic on the surface. Answering the following questions can help you identify whether you experienced a break in a bond with a parent. If you answer yes to any of them, it is likely you went through the interrupted movement. Take the time to write down your answers—and push yourself to respond with more than a yes or no; if an answer is a yes, how old were you when it happened? What is your memory of it? If the event pre-dates your memory, what have you heard about it?

Was your mother anxious, depressed, or under severe stress when she was pregnant with you?

Were there any difficulties between your parents during the pregnancy?

Were there complications during the pregnancy or during your birth?

Did your mother experience postpartum depression?

Did you experience a trauma or a separation from a parent during your first three years of life?

Did either of your parents experience a trauma during your first three years of life?

Did your mother experience a miscarriage before you were born?

Did either of your parents experience the death of a child before you were born?

In order to heal the wound caused by the interruption, we must complete the movement. In other words, we must reach out and someone must reach back. But because of the fear of rejection that we carry within us, it can be impossible to muster the courage to do so. Because of this, I often guide my clients in practicing reaching out, so that they can finally complete the circle of love. In a constellation setting, I will ask the person representing the parent of the "constellee" to embrace him or her, then make small circles on the nape of their neck with their hands, gently and lovingly. This re-creates the movement of love that was disrupted between parent and child. We can also hold the right hand of our parent's representative and walk in circles together, symbolically closing the loop.

Outside the setting of a constellation, you can ask your parent to embrace you and make small circles on your neck with their hands. If either of you is not comfortable doing so, or if you simply prefer, you can ask another person whom you trust and feel safe with to do so. Finally, you can—should—practice doing this yourself. You can parent yourself; you can give yourself the gift of reaching out and reaching back, showing up for yourself, extending yourself grace, and being gentle with yourself. Rub your own neck in small circles until you feel peaceful inside. You can even lie down and, using a neck pillow or a neck hammock, allow your body to relax completely so that the pillows or hammock provide counter tension. The key is to feel supported and thus able to let go. The more willing we are to accept self-love and self-respect from our "inner mother," the easier it will be for us to come to a reconciliation.

CHAPTER 4

Enlightened Love

Order and Disorder

Taking ownership of your life is hard freaking work. So take a moment here to acknowledge that—and to acknowledge yourself and the hard work you're doing. The hurt our parents may have caused is very real. That's exactly why we *start* with accepting them as the only right parents; dwelling first on *why* we reject our parents often leads to excuse making, a way of dodging leaning in, getting our hands dirty, and just doing the damn thing. And, of course, because the specificities of why are as unique as the individuals who experience them. But Family Constellations reveals that there *is* a universal why at the heart of rejection: a disorder in the family system.

In Family Constellations, we take great care in putting things in order. The family system *always* seeks order; if there is anything you've learned by now, it's that. The system always wants everything in its right place and every place filled. When things—*people*—are either not in place or out of place, that's when all bets are off and the system goes haywire. Order is such an interesting concept, when we really unpack its layers of meaning. There is the first and most obvious meaning: the arrangement of things or people, in relation to each other, in a particular sequence or pattern. But then there's the more social meaning of order, the way we use it when we talk about "law and order" or "calling a meeting to order" or even in describing a religious order—order as a set of rules that govern how a group operates, and the state of things when those rules are followed (in order). We've mostly been talking about order in the first sense, but family systems rely on both types of order: the order of people in a certain sequence and in specific places or roles in relation to each other, and the order of the rules that develop out of the sequence and which allow the system to function.

One of the—maybe *the*—fundamental governing rules, or orders, of the family system is the right to belong. When it comes to parents and children, ensuring and protecting a child's belonging is the fundamental role of the parent. It is the parent's responsibility to guarantee that a child feels secure in their belonging. They do this by communicating, in word and action, three bedrock promises:

- I see you.
- I hear you.
- I recognize you.

I see you means seeing a child for who they are: a child. Doing this means allowing a child to take his or her rightful place in the family system. Children should never become surrogates for an adult missing in a parent's life, especially a partner. Parents who treat their children as confidantes are not seeing their children. Parents who rely on their children for emotional support are not seeing their children. Parents who say, "My child is my best friend" are not seeing their child. Did I piss you off with that last one? It has become de rigueur for millennial parents to describe their children this way, but the thing is: Your child is not your friend. Children rely on their parents to survive. Children rely on their parents for social-emotional structure. Children rely on their parents to develop the skills they need to become functioning adults. These are not the needs of a friend. Finally, friends choose each other. Our children don't get to choose us, nor do we get to choose them, which so many people seem to forget—but more on that in a minute. When we refuse to allow our children to take their *rightful* place in the family system, we are excluding them from belonging.

I hear you means listening to your child, being emotionally available to your child. It means accepting the reality of a child's vast array of emotions and feelings, of actually listening to them as they tell us, in so many ways, what they need from us. When you tell a child he or she is "too sensitive," you're really telling them their feelings are an inconvenience for you. When you constantly play on your phone as your child vies for your attention, you're signaling clearly where your priorities lie. When you dismiss your child's fears, you teach them that they're not worthy of being taken seriously. Eventually, children who are not heard learn to silence themselves or to behave in negative ways that will secure attention. A silenced child is a child who has been excluded.

I recognize you means seeing a child as an individual person and supporting that individual as they are. Children are not an extension of their parents, which too many of us—and our own parents—forget. They are not there to fulfill a parent's own unmet goals or dreams. They are not there to bolster a parent's ego. We don't get to choose who they are or who they are going to become. We can help shape their emerging personhood through supportive guidance, but we are not here to mold them in our preferred image. Parents who require their children to be a certain kind of person, especially around gender expression and, later, sexuality, are erasing their child's identity. This erasure is another way that children experience a lack of belonging.

Disorder (and, eventually, rejection) happens when parents fail to meet their children's needs to be seen, heard, and recognized—to belong. Because, regardless of how they're treated, despite—or because of—how they're excluded, children will do anything to belong to their families. Children are fiercely loyal, especially and above all to their parents. It's a kind of loyalty that goes beyond self-preservation, though, a dangerous and potentially self-annihilating blind love or "crazy love" that does not necessarily serve their highest good, a love that causes children to subsume themselves—their own fate and destiny—to that of their parents. As Bert Hellinger wrote, "For a child, the worst thing that could possibly happen is to be shut out of the family. That's very fundamental. Children live in the awareness that they belong in their families; it's where they want to belong, and they share the fate of their families, whatever that fate may be. Therefore, children will do anything to protect that belonging, totally without regard for self."[3]

For my client George, his inner child's loyalty to his father had become an obstacle to his own happiness in adulthood. When George was just two years old, his mother left his father, and it would be nine years before George saw her again. George became his father's "best pal," his "little man," to whom he would complain ceaselessly about women, whom he described as crazy, drama-seeking, and untrustworthy, among other choice adjectives. George quickly learned never to express any interest in his mother—where she might be, what she was doing, or if he would ever hear from her again. He learned especially to never show sadness; when he did, his dad would "jokingly" say, "What's wrong, little man, ain't I enough for you? Don't worry, we don't need your mom; we've got each other."

In leaning on George for emotional support and in discussing his love life with him (especially in transmitting sexist and toxic generalizations about women), George's father was creating deep disorder in their home. He did not *see* George—who was a child—instead viewing him as a suitable confidant for adult matters. And he did not *hear* George, who learned to silence himself preemptively rather than give life to any feelings that might inconvenience his father. George did not feel secure in belonging to his family system; at a deep level, he felt rejected by his father, who refused to see or hear him.

As an adult, George struggled in romantic relationships with women. He was needy and co-dependent but also constantly tested the women in his life, inevitably driving them away. After a breakup, he would become obsessed with "getting revenge" on his ex, posting performative pictures on social media and competing with them mentally. He had never been in a relationship that lasted longer than a few months. George was self-aware enough to realize that the problem lay within him, rather than in the women he dated, *but* . . . he traced all of his issues back to his mother. Meanwhile, his dad was his "hero," his "rock," and his "best friend."

Together, George and I did a lot of inner child work in relationship to his mother, reconciling him to the reality that his mother had done the best she could and that leaving him had been an act of love because she had been unable to take care of him. He accepted her as his only right mother. We started with George's mother because that relationship *did* need healing; George *did* need to stop rejecting her in order to fully receive and be open to life. But we also started there because George was so resistant to seeing his father as anything less than perfect; his belonging rested on sharing his father's fate. It wasn't until George's anger and resentment toward his mother began to ebb that he became open to acknowledging what was with his father. This new openness wasn't even something he was necessarily aware of—but in a breakthrough constellation, George found himself taking a place next to his father, rather than in front of him. He could see the disorder immediately and no longer cared to deny it. As George took his rightful place in front of his father, the place of the child, his shoulders visibly relaxed, even as his spine straightened. "I feel so much . . . lighter," he told me. "I am your son, not your friend," he told his father. "I don't need to sabotage my own relationships to prove my loyalty to you. I don't need to share your fate."

After George's breakthrough with his dad, he decided to stop dating for the time being and to focus on getting to know himself. He realized that he was so enmeshed with his dad, he didn't really know what he wanted out of life, let alone relationships. He stopped seeing his mother as a villain and his father as a hero and allowed them to be just regular people with regular feelings, in other words, human—finally empowering himself to grant himself the same grace.

AFFIRMATIONS

I am seen; I am heard; I am recognized. I belong.

I have a place; I have a voice; I am my own person.

I am here to travel my own path.

EXERCISE: The Order of Love—Nurturing Belonging

Something I've witnessed with so many clients—and have experienced myself—is how desire for belonging often continues to drive us in adulthood, especially if we experienced its lack in our childhoods. Whether it is with our friends, at work, or especially with romantic partners, we seek to feel seen, heard, and recognized—and are often disappointed. What I've come to learn is that in our adult relationships, that sense of being understood and deeply valued for who we truly are comes only when we extend the same grace to others. When we see, hear, and recognize those who are central to our lives, we deepen our connection with them. It's through these authentic and meaningful connections that we find belonging.

This exercise is all about becoming better at making others feel seen and heard, primarily through deep listening. It's something you can do any time you're in conversation with someone else, whether that's talking to your long-distance best friend over FaceTime, playing make-believe with a child, sitting over mugs of tea at the kitchen table with a parent, meeting with co-workers at the conference table in your office, or lying in bed with a romantic partner.

LOOK UP: Seeing, hearing, and recognizing others begins with being present for them. It's impossible to recognize when someone is making a bid for connection—trying to secure your attention, affection, or acceptance verbally or nonverbally—when you're distracted by devices or your own thoughts. Put down your phone when you're spending time with someone else, especially when they're speaking. This may seem obvious, but so few people seem capable of doing so.

MAKE EYE CONTACT: Okay, you've put your phone away—huzzah! But now actually *look* at the person you're with. Don't stare out a window while they're talking, at another person across the room, or at your hands while you fiddle with a loose thread on your jeans. You don't have to maintain an unbroken stare (that would be creepy), but you know, seeing someone begins with seeing them.

LISTEN WITHOUT A MOTIVE: When you are really listening to someone, you are hearing what they are saying and simply absorbing it, without playing out your response in your head. Don't plan a rebuttal or start thinking about how they're missing the point, why they're wrong, or, heck, even why they're right. Once you're doing this, you're not listening anymore. The only conversation you're engaged in is the one you're having with yourself.

DON'T INTERRUPT: That's it. That's all I have to say here. Just don't f-ing interrupt. So simple, yet so hard.

ACKNOWLEDGE AND REFLECT: When the person is done speaking, acknowledge what they've said by reflecting it back to them. Do not make this about yourself. Many people mistake this as demonstrating empathy, but it mostly just feels self-centered. If your friend is talking to you about losing their job and how biased their boss was, you might say, "It's so unfair to be fired after all the work you've put in just because your boss plays favorites." Do not say, "When I had a shitty boss who forced me out so he could hire his son-in-law, I felt so angry too."

ALLOW YOUR FRIEND/FAMILY MEMBER/COLLEAGUE/PARTNER THEIR FEELINGS: Don't try to downplay, fix, or rescue the situation. When we do this, it's often because of our own discomfort with someone else's negative feelings or pain, even if we believe we're just trying to help. When we try to "make things better," we are basically broadcasting that we aren't really there for the person in that moment; it's all about us again and how we feel. After you've acknowledged and reflected back what they've said, you can try asking something like, "Are you in a place right now where you really just need to talk through what's happening, or do you want to talk about what comes next?"

Sheltering the Inner Child

For many of us, that "anything" a child will do to protect his or her belonging means not only "accepting" not being seen, heard, or recognized—consciously or unconsciously adapting ourselves to meet our parents' needs—but unconsciously taking on our parents' pain, as well, in the innocent belief that we can carry it for them. We believe that if we can shoulder the burden, they will be relieved and order will be restored, reinstating our belonging (or theirs, in the case of an excluded parent). We try to fix our parents' unhappiness by suffering for them. In this way, entanglements always show us where our loyalty—and love—lies, even if we believe, as my client Jonathan did, that we feel nothing for a parent or consciously feel antipathy toward them. We become entangled with our parents *because of our loyalty to them*, which is a form of blind love.

But the belief that we can absolve someone else of their fate, or at least share it with them, is a kind of fantasy, particular to the arrogance of childhood, in which we think we know better than our parents. It is a naive and, well, childish form of magical thinking. And in indulging this fantasy, children violate one of the basic orders of life itself: Parents give, and children receive. In fact, the most frequent family disorder issue I have witnessed in Family Constellations—as a facilitator, representative, or observer—is when the child takes care of his mother/father and becomes the adult, while the adult becomes the child.

And we know where that leads. But we're grown-ups now, right? Not children. We know better, don't we? Well . . . *sort of.* Most of us understand how profoundly our childhoods shape who we become. It's easy to make the connection between the overt values transmitted to us (like religious or political beliefs) or the particular socioeconomic circumstances of our families and our adult attitudes toward education, career, or family, for example. But few of us are attuned to the ongoing existence of our inner child—that part of our personality that feels and reacts to life the way a child does—or are aware of how much it continues to inform and direct our choices and behaviors. Our inner child remains loyal. That's not only why we repeat our parents' mistakes and misfortunes but also why so few people do better than their parents: because to do so would feel like a form of betrayal.

Our inner child remains wounded until we do the work of healing. The thing is, healing begins by accepting that we can't change other people and we can't rescue them. There is a profound loss involved in accepting this, though. Bert Hellinger put it beautifully when he described suffering with a problem as "easier to bear than a resolution" because "suffering and continuing to carry a problem are deeply bound to a feeling of innocence and loyalty. . . . It is the deep hope that through one's own suffering, another person will be rescued."[4] No one can heal his or her parents. The only person we can heal is ourselves. This is an important gift that we make to our family as well. Because by healing ourselves, we offer a space of healing for the next generations.

When my client Leslie's inner child finally accepted that she could not rescue her mother, she experienced deep healing—but she also mourned. Leslie was 43 when we started working together. She was 13 years into a marriage that had been unhappy for at least 10 of them. As Leslie described her husband's habits of belittling and demeaning her, it seemed clear to me that he was verbally and emotionally abusive—though Leslie never used that language. Instead, she focused on how they needed to improve their communication. Leslie characterized herself as strong and indicated that her strength intimidated her husband and that was the reason for his "outbursts." Leslie's strength was in stark contrast to her mother, as she depicted her. Leslie pitied her mother (and seemed to resent her), who had stayed with Leslie's abusive father until Leslie was 13. "By the end, my dad assaulted my mom at least once a week—it got worse over the years," Leslie said. "But it wasn't until he pulled a gun on her that she left him. All that time, I had to take care of my little sister. I had to protect her. I had to shield her from what was going on. My mom was a shell of a person; she did the bare minimum for us. I swore I would never be like her. That's why I'm so strong. I don't take shit from anyone."

But Leslie *was* taking on the burden of her mother's pain, whether she could see it or not. Though Leslie initially portrayed her husband's behavior as "frustrating," it became clear that Leslie walked on eggshells around him, trying to preempt and stave off his outbursts. She often explained to me why, even though her husband's response was "a little over the top," she *was* at fault in some way for whatever he was blaming her for. And her sense of self-worth was in the gutter. She had unwittingly come to believe all the nasty insults she'd been pelted with: that she was stupid, thoughtless, selfish, and unattractive. Leslie was in an abusive relationship. It may not have become physically abusive, like her mother's, but nonetheless, she was in a marriage that was turning her into "a shell of a person." And her identity as a "strong woman," seemingly assembled from a pastiche of inspirational quotes and mostly exhibited at work and in her social life (though she said friends had told her she was "abrasive"), was more a shield protecting herself from the truth than anything.

It didn't escape my notice that Leslie had decided to seek help 13 years into her marriage—just as her mother had mustered the courage to exit her marriage when Leslie was 13. Leslie's inner child, her little girl, was fully aligned with her mama. In entering and staying in an abusive relationship, Leslie was taking on the fate of her mother and attempting to rewrite her mother's destiny through her own story—trying to rescue her. In constellation,

Leslie embraced her seated "mother," trying to help her stand. When Leslie and her mother switched places, Leslie began to cry. Finally, when Leslie was ready to stand, her mother took her place behind Leslie. "It was like when I was sitting in the chair, I was a child again. And I finally let myself truly feel my fear and sadness that, as a kid, I worked so hard to suppress just to survive. It was like I told my little girl, 'It's okay to be sad and scared. You don't have to pretend anymore. I'll take care of you.' And when I stood up and my mom took her rightful place, I was finally really an adult." In accepting her mother's love and giving her mother her right place, Leslie found that her anger and resentment gave way to empathy. Leslie's anger had shielded her from having to overtly acknowledge the desperation and fear her mother had felt. When empathy flooded in, Leslie experienced deep sorrow for her mother. She was no longer reacting as her inner child, whom she was now caring for, but as an adult who had given up the fantasy that she could right the wrongs of the past.

The challenge of healing is to learn to acknowledge the inner child, get to know her, accept her, and love her. As an adult, our role is to promise our inner child: *I see you; I hear you; I recognize you.* One of the best ways we can keep these promises to our inner child is by moving from *blind love* to *enlightened love* when it comes to our families, especially to our parents. The inner child experiences blind love; a fully realized adult transitions to enlightened love. When we love blindly, we sacrifice our own highest good in order to belong. We don't see people for who they are, and we don't—can't—see reality as it is. We reject or we idealize. With blind love, we are driven by fear and obligation. When love is enlightened, we don't sacrifice our higher good to placate or please others. We make choices that are in integrity with our values and in so doing, we best support others. *We see people for who they are, without judgment;* we are able to acknowledge not only their flaws but also what they have given us. We accept reality and we accept what is beyond our power to control: other people.

The key to enlightened love is setting boundaries. When you set boundaries, you tacitly acknowledge that the only person you can control is yourself. Setting boundaries is a way of taking agency in your life. A boundary is in its literal sense a limit. It's a line or border that separates one place from another. A boundary marks the place where one person ends and another begins. A boundary is a line you don't cross, and a line you enforce others from crossing. When you lack boundaries, you allow others to determine how you think, act, and feel. Your sense of your own identity apart from the wants and needs of others may be weak. When you set boundaries, however, you draw a clear line between what you are willing to accept and what you are not, between what belongs to you and what does not, such as responsibility for someone else's feelings. When you set boundaries, you create space for yourself, a space that is inviolate and in which you have the freedom to assess who you are and how you want to be, especially in relation to other people. It may seem like setting boundaries will separate you from other people, but healthy boundaries engender respect and actually improve relationships, bringing you closer rather than farther apart.

Finding the right distance between yourself and your parents—setting your limits—is both literally and metaphorically the only way to gain perspective. When you're not used to it, though, setting boundaries can feel, oddly, like a transgression. But think of it this way: In healthy families, children learn to separate from their parents. Those earliest separations are a transgression of sorts. Children start lying around two or three, and this is a good thing; it's one of the earliest indicators that they understand the difference between themselves and mom or dad, that they have their own interiority that is inaccessible to their parents. In adolescence we test our boundaries even further, missing curfew, dating someone our parents don't approve of, smoking cigarettes or trying alcohol—as we hurtle toward cutting the cord; loving parents celebrate these tests even as they worry, because it means their child is moving toward independence. And independence requires boundaries between parent and child. Hellinger underscored the healthiness of the adolescence crisis when he wrote, "Every child has to overstep the rules in order to continue developing. That's how progress is made. The parents forbid something because they feel it's necessary to do so, but secretly they often hope that the child will disobey the restriction."[5]

My client Rachel described her family as "really close-knit" and "very loving." She was 24 and spoke with her parents every single day, although she lived in New York and they lived in Florida. Rachel came to me because she was struggling with severe anxiety—the smallest decisions had started to paralyze her; she was constantly afraid of making the wrong choice, believing that a disastrous outcome lurked just around the corner of every decision. "My parents are obsessed with safety," she told me, "so that's probably part of it; like, they have cameras *everywhere*, so I guess I'm just naturally oriented toward being paranoid and risk averse."

As I would come to learn, Rachel didn't just grow up with parents obsessed with safety—her safety (and her younger brother's) in particular was one of their primary fixations. Every decision Rachel made about her life had to be vetted by her parents: what she studied, what kind of work she did, where she worked, where she lived, who she dated. They chose her doctors. When Rachel left Florida after college to pursue her career in New York, her parents had insisted she live on the Upper East Side rather than in Brooklyn, where all of her friends lived. As a result, Rachel felt socially isolated and lonely—seeing her friends meant an hour-plus subway ride each way or a very hefty cab fare; they were rarely willing to schlep across the East River and then uptown.

But Rachel was 24, right? Why didn't she just do what she wanted? The answer was a bit complicated, especially to Rachel, who had never considered the question. "I'm not really here because of an issue with my parents," she reminded me. "I'm just hoping to figure out the source of my constant anxiety and fear. My parents are super supportive." *Supportive* being the key word—Rachel's parents, who were quite wealthy, supported her financially. They paid her rent, they paid her bills, they paid for her groceries; they even deposited "fun money" in her account every month. If Rachel didn't do what they wanted, they would withhold funds. They controlled Rachel financially. Even if they did it from a place of love, as they (and she) believed, it was still control. They didn't recognize Rachel as an individual; instead, she was an extension of her parents, another piece of property to be monitored and safeguarded.

Rachel's parents had made every decision for her for so long that Rachel had very little sense of what she really wanted. As a result, she was deeply alienated from who she was, independent of them. She had no identity of her own. She didn't know how to *be*. When she did make choices that she knew they wouldn't approve of—like whom she planned on voting for in the presidential election—she kept it a secret, which increased her anxiety.

It was ironic: Rachel's parents' need to keep Rachel safe had actually led to her feeling deeply unsafe, because she had no boundaries. She not only had no boundaries with her parents, but she had also never learned to set boundaries in general, as a result of her parents' dominance over her life. When we don't have healthy boundaries, we naturally feel unsafe—there is no border between us and others, nothing to prevent others from trespassing in our lives. Rachel's intense anxiety was a direct by-product of her parents' "support." Her anxiety had begun when she moved to New York and continued to grow because, for the first time ever, she had to rely on her own judgment—in which she had little to no confidence—at least part of the time. Rachel didn't trust herself; she didn't feel safe with herself. Rachel didn't value herself; her value came from pleasing her parents.

As Rachel came to terms with the way her parents' need to control her had obliterated her sense of identity and squashed her spirit, she became deeply angry and resentful. Her first impulse was to cut them out of her life completely, to go no-contact. Rejection. And it made sense—Rachel's inner child felt rejected and wanted to strike back. Instead, we talked about how, after she accepted her parents as her only right parents, we could truly serve her inner child. How could Rachel re-parent herself? How could she come to recognize herself?

Rachel determined that as difficult and frightening as it might be, she needed to set a firm boundary with her parents regarding money. She stopped taking it from them. It was difficult, and it was frightening. But in doing so, Rachel began having to set other boundaries—she began having to learn what she would and would not tolerate, what she valued, what she would and would not compromise in service to those values. Budgeting meant picking and choosing—her food, her clothes, even her friends. Who would stand by her when she was no longer footing the bill for a night out? Would she still accept sexist, subpar treatment at work, now that slower promotions meant living paycheck to paycheck for another year or three? Now that she was no longer cushioned—you might even say anesthetized—by the soft landing of her parents' money, what did she really care about?

Rachel's friendships deepened. She switched tracks in her industry. She started cooking for herself (delivery was no longer an everyday option) and discovered a hobby that she became passionate about. She started dating—something that had seemed too daunting in the past, when any boyfriend would have to meet with her parents' approval. She no longer shared every detail of her life with her parents, no longer turned to them for advice at every critical juncture. And, at first, Rachel's relationship with her parents did suffer. They were hurt; they felt angry and rejected. But as Rachel continued to meet them with enlightened love and to demonstrate her competence at life, as she continued to build trust in herself, they began to trust in her too.

Ultimately, rejection is a defense mechanism. Though in the end it may be a strategy that harms us more than it helps us, it is a completely understandable reaction to pain caused by our parents. Because in relation to our parents, our inner child is calling the shots. And children have very few ways to fend for themselves without adult protection. But we *are* adults, and we can offer our inner child that protection. We *can* parent our inner child ourselves. We can, and we must, shelter our inner child.

AFFIRMATIONS

I cannot change, fix, or rescue others.

Choosing my highest good is an act of love.

I give myself permission to take care of myself.

EXERCISE: Setting Boundaries

Most of us struggle with setting boundaries due to fear. We might fear losing a relationship, hurting someone's feelings, being perceived as difficult, or forgoing validation or approval. Essentially, we fear rejection—losing our belonging. In early childhood we internalize lessons about boundaries, mostly from our parents. When there is disorder in our family system, we learn quickly that having porous boundaries—when we subsume our own needs in favor of others'—can secure our belonging. When we attempt to set boundaries in adulthood, our inner child might panic. They might insist that disaster looms. They might try to wheedle, beg, or negotiate their way out of drawing that line in the sand. But remember: You are a grown-up now. The most caring thing you can do for your inner child is to be the parent, *be the adult*. Shelter them, keep them safe, and help them become secure in themselves by showing them that you *really* see them, hear them, and recognize them. Do this by setting boundaries, boundaries that reinforce *what* you see, hear, and recognize. In other words, respond to *your* needs and values first, rather than those of others.

Boundaries can be rigid, porous, or healthy—while we're always aiming for the last one, many of us grapple with the first two in at least some area of our lives. Rigid boundaries are boundaries that are too inflexible; they are boundaries that have become more like walls, defense mechanisms designed to prevent the intrusion of anything perceived as threatening. Rigid boundaries prevent growth and intimacy. Porous boundaries are boundaries that are too permeable; they are boundaries that are easily dismantled or overcome, where the distinction between self and other is obscured or erased. When your boundaries are porous, you allow others to make decisions for you, implicitly or explicitly.

There are many different types of boundaries: physical (your boundaries around your body), emotional (your boundaries around your feelings), intellectual (your boundaries around your thoughts and ideas), material (boundaries around money and possessions), and boundaries around time (your use of it and how others expect you to spend it), among others. The degree to which you feel comfortable enforcing those various boundaries will of course differ; you might generally have healthy physical boundaries but porous intellectual ones. And when and how you exercise any one boundary also depends on context; the nature of your boundaries will likely shift between settings (in a work meeting versus at brunch with friends) and between people, varying when dealing with friends versus family members versus colleagues versus romantic partners, etc.

Again, setting boundaries isn't easy; I won't pretend that it is. But I don't need to—because you've got this. Like any hard thing, it gets easier with repetition and time. When it comes to getting comfortable asserting yourself, start small. Practice setting low-stakes boundaries at first—each success fuels your bravery for more challenging situations. A low-stakes boundary might mean saying no to someone you already trust and have a healthy relationship with (e.g., someone who doesn't balk at not getting their way). Maybe this is a good friend who asks you to dinner. When they suggest a restaurant that you can't afford, say no. Rather than agreeing, then spending the night anxious and resentful about how much it's costing you, try saying something like, "I can't wait to see you. Chez Louis is out of my budget right now. How about Joe's?" Your friend's likely normal reaction (remember, I did say pick someone you trust . . . in other words, someone who isn't a self-centered a-hole) will be the small victory that empowers you to take on bigger challenges. Ready to start?

DEFINE YOUR BOUNDARIES: The first step in setting boundaries is knowing what your boundaries are. A good way to get in touch with them is to start by being radically honest with yourself about what you need and want out of any given relationship, be it with your mother or with your boss. Take the time to write this down. Next, focus on your rights and values. By "rights," I mean the fundamental rights we each have simply by being born—the right to bodily autonomy, the right to be free from harm, the right to express our feelings without fear of judgment, for example. List what you feel those rights are. Finally, home in on your values. Make a list of them: Aim for 15 or 20, then narrow it to 10, then 5. Reading through those values, ask yourself if, when, and to what degree you are willing to compromise on those values. Now look back over what you've written regarding what you need and want. How does the relationship meet or fail to meet those needs? Does the relationship honor your rights? Are you able to be in integrity with your values in this relationship? Answering these questions can help you identify where you need to draw better boundaries.

COMMIT TO YOUR BOUNDARIES: Commit to putting your own needs first. Commit to keeping your responsibilities in sight: You are responsible for your feelings, your choices, and your behaviors; you are not responsible for the feelings, choices, and behaviors of others. Commit to being okay with yourself; your well-being is not dependent on the validation and approval of others. Commit to ceding attempts at control; you cannot fix, rescue, or save other people. Set consequences for violations of boundaries and follow through on them. Plan for and accept possible negative outcomes of setting boundaries, such as the possibility that you may anger and upset those who are used to steamrolling you. Doing so makes it easier to overcome your fear, follow through, and stay committed.

COMMUNICATE YOUR BOUNDARIES: Speak up, first and foremost, preferably before someone has a chance to violate your boundaries (again). Express yourself clearly, calmly, and without hesitation. This means being direct (don't beat around the bush), assertive (be confident), *and* respectful (not accusatory or aggressive). Say no without ambiguity. "No" is a complete sentence. Address why the boundary is important to you and the consequences for violating it. Keep the focus on yourself—this isn't about the other person's behavior (which you can't control) or about punishing them. For example, if you need to set a time boundary with a co-worker, you might say, "I respond to e-mails only during work hours," rather than "Don't e-mail me after work hours." If you're setting boundaries with a family member, you might say, "It's important to me that I feel heard in conversation. If I feel like I'm being interrupted or spoken over, I'll exit the conversation," rather than "If you interrupt me while we're talking, I'm going to stop speaking to you." Don't JADE—justify, argue, defend, or explain. You have the right to self-determination. In most interpersonal exchanges, if someone challenges your boundaries, you are not obligated to explain yourself (unless you're at work, where your job might depend on it), and you never need to apologize. When a person doesn't respect your boundaries and you still engage with them, you validate the possibility that there is a good reason to question your boundary. There isn't.

Precedence and Priority

This chapter was *almost* called "The Orders of Love," a reference to Hellinger's concept that the family system is ruled by three orders—meaning order as a set of rules that govern how the system operates—that function almost like natural laws. These orders, when complied with, allow love (enlightened love) to flow freely within the family system and forward on to the next generations. We've been diving into these orders all along, though I've never explicitly called them out as such—the less jargon, the better. But since we're all about order and disorder now, let's get into it. You're ready for the heady stuff.

You've got the first order of love down by now: *belonging* (i.e., everyone has the right to belong). The second order of love is *balance*: everyone in their place. The third order of love, well, that one can seem a little arbitrary on its surface: It's *precedence*. Precedence? Basically, in relationship dynamics within the family, it means who comes first has priority. It's the sequence part of order we talked about earlier. Parents (and their relationship) take priority over children, children have priority over parents' new partners, older siblings have priority over younger siblings (don't worry, younger siblings, it doesn't mean your parents love you less or owe you less—just trust me for now), etc. First come, first served. Precedence tells us who has priority. This is one of the ways that we know our place.

Priority doesn't mean a certain family member deserves better treatment or *more* attention, however. Instead, priority means knowing how to appropriately direct our attention. A disregard or lack of respect for priority in the family system is one of the greatest threats to its order and central to the dysfunctional dynamics so many of us grew up in—and now risk perpetuating ourselves. While our relationship to our parents is the primary family dynamic we experience, secondary family dynamics, such as our parents' relationship to each other, the presence of stepparents, our sibling bonds (or lack thereof), and adoption, among others, are often a hot mess of skewed priorities that block the free flow of love in the family system, creating a deep well of disorder.

As children, our relationship to our parents or caregivers is the most central and most overwhelming relationship we experience. But critical to the quality of that relationship is our parents' relationship (or lack thereof) with each other. Parents come before children. That is the order of precedence. Two people must literally first join their genetic material in order to create a new human. The child comes after this union. Precedence tells us that this relationship has priority over the parents' relationship to the child. This might seem anathema to you, especially in our culture, which celebrates a sort of cultish devotion to one's children. *Of course, your child should come first!* you might be thinking. Anything else would be unforgivably selfish. When we think about priority as a tool for directing our attention appropriately, however, it's easier to understand. Children want to feel secure. They feel secure when their home life feels secure, when they take for granted and don't have to question the strength of the bond between their parents—this is safety for a child. Parents who focus on the quality of their relationship with each other, who nurture and sustain their love and commitment, create a loving environment for their child. Prioritizing your partner does not mean failing to attend to the needs of your child or treating them as secondary. It's quite the opposite: In prioritizing your partner, you are actually simultaneously valuing your child's well-being. For a child, becoming the primary relationship of a parent can be deeply damaging. Not only does this tend to lead to instability in the home (e.g., a failed relationship between the parents), but it can create in children an unfair sense of obligation or debt to that parent, a guilty sense that the child owes them in return: be it attention, time, love, etc. Children are not and never should be indebted to their parents. The gift of life is impossible to repay; it can only be paid forward.

Of course, children can be and are happy in single-parent homes. I'm not saying that children require two parents in the same home (or even two parents at all) to be well-adjusted and to thrive. I am saying that there must be respect between parents. Even parents who split must continue to prioritize the health of their relationship before that of their children. It's an oft-repeated statistic that 50 percent of marriages end in divorce. Yeah, the number is anecdotal, but our willingness to accept it as fact points to how common and how normalized divorce is in our society. But just because something is common doesn't mean it lacks impact. Yes, most children whose parents divorce are better off than they would be living in the midst of a miserable relationship. But divorce is still a huge moment in the life of a child—it's the end of something they viewed almost as a fact of nature, a sudden shift in reality, a transition to a new way of living and relating. Unfortunately, so many adults who share children handle their breakup in the shittiest ways possible, with overt acrimony, bitterness, and bile, with total disrespect for the ex-relationship . . . the relationship that produced the child or children. Too often the adults' storm sweeps up the children. The parents ask them to choose their camp, either overtly or covertly. They are put in the middle of this war and are expected to be a counselor or a mediator, which is inappropriate and devastating.

Prioritizing the parental relationship in a divorce does not mean our parents can't or shouldn't experience anger and hurt, especially in the wake of an abusive relationship. It doesn't mean a parent has to like his or her ex, even a little. People end up with shitty partners. Even though in almost all relationships, both parties bear some responsibility for its dissolution, that responsibility might only be one percent. When you're leaving someone who bears 99 percent of the responsibility for the breakdown of your relationship, how could you possibly prioritize the relationship with them? You do it by ending the relationship with respect for your story and all it encompasses, especially and including your children, who carry elements of both parents within. My mentor, Suzi Tucker, teaches that "rejecting the other parent is rejecting the other parent inside the child." If we don't accept an ex-partner with love and respect, how can we imagine that we can properly love and accept our children as they are? As with a parent, when we reject a partner with whom we created a child (rather than accept the reality of who they are, without judgment and with enlightened love), we reject life itself: the life of the child and the gift of life they carry within from that partner.

The family system will stay the same in a divorce. While a divorce spells the end of a love story between the parents, the love for the children should not be questioned. The family system will always provide a safe platform for the children if the parents remain together inside the children, that is, if parents remain active in their roles as mother and father and keep their children out of the divorce. They are and will always be "together" for their children as a pairing. Regarding their coupling as a man and woman in marriage, it is their own business and has to stay that way. Here, Suzi Tucker advises: "If the parents include each other even as they withdraw from one another, the children have an easier transition." Ultimately, a child must not interfere in the parents' affairs. Parents have to bear their own choices. We must stand in our role, as the child, and focus on our own future, so that we don't live in theirs. As Bert Hellinger said, "Divorce is a matter between the parents and it's not the children's business."

Following divorce, many people remarry or re-partner. The entrance of a stepparent into the life of a child is often messy at best and painful at worst, both for the child and the stepparent. Merging two families—balancing two existing family systems— is no easy task. Understanding our place, and the role of others, in this new dynamic is confusing and disorienting. An individual's children from a previous partnership obviously precede the new relationship: They take precedence and have priority. Or they should, in theory. Unfortunately, parents often have to contend with two sets of seemingly competing needs, two sets of insecurities: the new partner who wants to be reassured of their importance, and the child who wants to be reassured of their parent's loyalty. The archetype of the wicked stepmother, deeply ingrained in our cultural psyche, illustrates this deep-seated fear centered on being replaced and left unprotected by a parent who is choosing a new family. But when both child and stepparent can inhabit their rightful place in the family system, when precedence and priority are respected, both feel more secure and are able to be open to each other. A child who feels their parent's unwavering commitment to them can rest in that trust. They trust that their parent will not choose the stepparent over them and no longer view the stepparent as competition. They are open to the stepparent and to a healthy relationship of mutual respect.

Similarly, a stepparent who fully accepts, understands, and supports his or her partner's commitment to their child creates a relationship with their partner that is stronger, more loving, and better bonded. A stepparent who does not overstep bounds and who respects and honors the child's biological father or mother also creates a better bond with their stepchild. Stepparents who speak poorly of a partner's ex or otherwise demonstrate disdain inadvertently subject a child to a loyalty test, which the stepparent is bound to lose. Remember, children are loyal to their parents. Even a positive relationship with a stepparent can feel like a betrayal to a child. When we allow a child to rest assured that we are not a threat to the other parent, we ease their potential burden of guilt.

Even if our parents split when we're no longer children, the dissolution of their marriage and introduction of subsequent new relationships can be deeply unsettling. During one of the classes I took when studying to become a Family Constellations facilitator, the teacher taught a daylong unit on blended families—stepparents, stepsiblings, and half siblings. At the beginning of the class, she asked us to raise our hands if we had stepparents. I had no idea how to answer. In that moment, I realized with surprising force how uncertain my footing in my family system really was. I had been focused on my relationship with my father, but I had to face the fact that my relationship with my mother—whom, as you know by now, I idolized—was not as straightforward as I liked to imagine.

My parents divorced when I was 22, so they had already raised me into adulthood by that stage and, in theory, taught me everything I needed to know. The job was done. My mother remarried two years later. I didn't actively dislike my mother's new husband, but I had no interest in getting to know him. Just none, which was maybe a bit churlish. I bristled at the thought of calling him my stepfather. From my perspective, my mother's new husband was only a part of the new partnership they set up together, which I had nothing to do with. I didn't live at home; hell, I didn't even live in the same country. In my view, he was not part of my *family*.

My mother wanted us to eventually relate as family, however. I resented this deeply. Privately, I felt my mother had imploded the perfectly fine family I'd already had. And even though I was supposedly an adult, I felt rejected—as though she had chosen a new life over her old life, meaning me. Yet I still felt guilty about my hesitation. I wanted to know if my behavior toward her husband (studied indifference) was okay, or if I had to make some adjustments. I explained my situation to my teacher. Her answer was crystal clear, and it helped me to accept him. "He is not your stepfather," she told me. "He is your mom's partner. She looks at you with this man at her side. Find a way to open your heart to his heart so that you include him in your private sphere, with healthy boundaries."

Realizing I did not have to accept my mother's husband as my stepfather softened me to accepting him as my mother's partner. That was a dynamic I was able to make room for, and in doing so, I could step back into my first position, as my mother's daughter. This simple approach worked perfectly for me and brought me peace regarding my mother's new relationship.

When parents divorce and remarry after a child is on their own, that generally means the new partner won't be a stepparent in the everyday sense. We are already on our own path. Treating the new partner as a stepparent can introduce disorder in our family system. We may be giving them a place that would or should best be occupied by another. We may use them to displace our feelings about a parent, whether negative or positive. In my case, I could have just as easily sought out a close relationship with my mother's husband in a misguided attempt to heal my relationship with my father.

Children who are adopted exist within a particularly complex family system—two systems, in fact—that relies especially heavily on respect for precedence and priority. To put it bluntly, adoptive parents must recognize that biological parents come first. Without them, there would be no child. Even though the biological parents lose their rights, they don't lose their place. Adoptive parents must respect and acknowledge the reality of the biological parents' existence (and of their ethnicity, race, and culture, when they differ from their own). Only then can they truly respect their child. When adoptive parents can say in their hearts, "Thanks to you, I became a parent," they create space for their child just as they are and they create space for the child's eventual acceptance of their adoption.

It's critical to share the truth with children, to tell them that they were adopted. We can't take away their fundamental right to their own origin story. If we do, how could we expect them to find their place or to fully acknowledge what is? A child who is adopted needs to consent to what the parents decided— to consent to reality. Only through this awareness and consent can an adopted child grow up serenely. When we lie to adopted children, we distort their reality. We steal part of their identity as we found our relationship with them on fear and insecurity. We create disorder.

When children are encouraged and allowed to love the reality of their biological parents openly, they are less likely to find covert, destructive ways to do so. And they are better equipped to understand that adoption was the adults' decision, a decision that in no way reflects on them or their worth, and in fact celebrates the value of their life. The child has no responsibility in the act of adoption and doesn't have to bear this choice or atone for the adults in their lives.

My client Michael didn't find out he was adopted until he was in his late teens. The revelation completely disoriented him, upending everything he thought he knew about his family and who he was fundamentally. On top of that, his parents' account of his adoption story was maddeningly vague. Michael's parents wouldn't tell him the name of the adoption agency they'd worked with or even where he'd been born. All he knew was that he'd been adopted in California, the most populous state in the country, where his parents had been living at the time. "It was a closed adoption for a reason," Michael's mother said. At an extremely critical moment in time—late adolescence, just as Michael was preparing to leave home and go to college—his trust in his parents was shattered, his stable foundation destroyed. In his late twenties, with the advent of DNA tracing sites like 23andMe, Michael decided to try and find any relatives on his own, frustrated with his parents' stonewalling. But what happened next further shook his sense of self-worth: He matched with a person who appeared to be his full biological sister. Same mother, same father. Michael would come to learn that his biological parents had stayed together after giving him up and had gone on to have another child, a daughter, whom they raised. After Michael reconnected with his sister, he learned that his biological parents had only revealed Michael's existence to her after she had become pregnant—she now had a baby boy. Michael, who had been an only child, felt both overjoyed to discover he had a sibling and also deeply rejected by his birth parents who had "given him away" but "kept" his sister.

Michael couldn't help but wonder what might have been different if both families had been truthful with their children. His whole life he had struggled with a feeling of not belonging, of shame, and with persistent depression. What if Michael's parents had told him the truth, had offered him his story, from earliest childhood? Michael felt he would have grown up perceiving his existence as the product of acts of love—love on the part of the people who strove to find a better life for him and love on the part of the people who wanted to give him that life—and that he would have felt greater self-acceptance and security, rather than less. His parents had worried that telling him he was adopted would make him feel bad—and that he might love them less. But instead their secrecy and silence had engendered an aura of there being something to hide.

Michael set to work sheltering his inner child immediately after we began working together. After meeting several times via video call, Michael set boundaries with his biological parents, who wanted to fast-forward into an intense family relationship that Michael wasn't ready for or even sure he wanted. He set boundaries with his parents, who wanted to know every detail of Michael's interactions with his biological family. He made clear to everyone that he was not interested in continuing a relationship that included lying. He and his sister did decide to meet, without any parents involved. In meeting his sister and nephew, Michael's deep healing began. Like him, she had been kept in the dark. Together, they shared their stories with each other, without acrimony, recrimination, or blame. It was a safe place to explore and talk about what had happened to them. Michael felt comfortable forging a connection with his sister, as she had played no part in his adoption. She, too, had been an only sibling, and had always felt a sense that "something"—or someone—was missing from her life. As Michael integrated his sibling—the only person who truly shared even a part of his strange fate—and his nephew into his life, he found himself more and more able to accept what was. As he gained empathy for his parents—their fears, their choices, and their fierce love—his anger ebbed. Finally, with respect for their fate and with enlightened love, he was able to accept both his biological mother and father and his adoptive parents as "the only right parents." Acceptance, as always, is the fastest way to move on and wholeheartedly live our life.

After the relationship with our parents, the most common intimate dynamic that most of us experience in childhood is our relationship with a sibling (even an only child is defined through the absence of a sibling). Regardless of how close we are or were with our siblings, they occupy a unique place in our lives that no one else can match: They are the only people with whom we share a real degree of our fate. Our brothers and our sisters are the only people who come into existence just as we did: through the shared lineage of our parents and our ancestors. They are often our longest-lasting relationship, too, eclipsing in duration any other bond.

As our first peers, our siblings become our earliest test subjects in our social experiments. The sibling relationship is where we learn to navigate so many of life's opposing and complementary dynamics: cooperation and competition, loyalty and antagonism, rivalry and teamwork, alliances and individualism. In adulthood, how we share and how we take our place in our environment can be traced back to those early dynamics.

Our siblings can be our best friends or our most loathed adversaries. Our siblings are primed to understand us as no one else can, but they are just as likely to misunderstand us more grievously than anyone else. This is because in childhood, our relationship with a sibling is never truly direct; how we see them is always mediated through our relationship to our parents, to our position in the family. The truth is, tensions with your siblings or sibling rivalry are never really about your brother or sister—they are always, in the end, about how your parents treated you. When we feel the need to compete with a sibling, we are competing for our parents' resources (time, attention, approval), no matter how old we are or whether or not our parents are still living.

So many parents make the mistake of comparing their children, even if inadvertently, rather than celebrating their distinct strengths. They may transfer their expectations from one child (who "failed" to meet them) to another. They may identify more with one child than another. The special needs of one child may simply require more of a parent's time. Parents may, indeed, have favorites. Favoritism is not what precedence-based priority is about. It does not mean that the firstborn child deserves more or better and that each child thereafter gets less (this isn't Regency England, after all). Not at all.

So, what could precedence and priority possibly mean when it comes to siblings, then? Well, so many of the issues we've just touched on are a violation of order, a failure to respect precedence and priority. How so? Again, I like to think of priority as knowing how to direct our attention appropriately. When we have multiple children, keeping precedence and priority in mind helps us meet the unique needs of our children, given their place in the family system. It means accurately seeing them in their rightful place, not comparing them. For example, an oldest child is the only sibling who ever experienced being the sole focus of his or her parents. He or she may more naturally take the lead. Unfavorably comparing a middle child, who may excel at brokering compromise, or a younger child, who may shine at securing a spotlight, to an oldest child is to resist the order of the family system—to disorder it.

You can't compare children when you understand that each is in the place they are meant to be. Parents who compare their children create disorder. When there *is* favoritism present, it's almost always a result of disorder in precedence. In a family where priority has been disordered and belonging is lacking, a parent might expect a child to take on the role of a younger or older sibling, causing strain, jealousy, and resentment between siblings. When parents uphold the order of precedence, they are better equipped to enforce belonging—to make sure that their children are seen, heard, and recognized.

As adults, we can choose to parent differently than our mother or father did, supporting order in our chosen families. But we can't go back in time and redo our parents' choices, nor can we control them in the present. Deepening sibling bonds, should you wish to, or simply letting go of poisonous resentments that harm you more than anyone else, begins with knowing and accepting your place. I don't mean this in the negative way people often wield the phrase "know your place," as a command to stay small, to not dream of more for yourself. I mean instead that you should come to truly understand the strengths of your unique place in your family system and celebrate it. Stop focusing on your sibling—it's not about how you're similar or different and why that's good or bad.

The fact is, you may never share the same perspective as a sibling. Ask any two siblings to recount the story of a shared family experience and you'll likely get two very different stories. Though you do share a large degree of fate with your siblings, at the same time, each child almost has a different set of parents. Perhaps when you were born, your parents were young and financially insecure, but when your sibling arrived they were older and had money. Perhaps when your sibling was born, your mother was still practicing law or medicine or teaching but decided to become a stay-at-home parent after your birth. Whatever the case may be, in this way, you and your sibling have very different fates. Respect theirs as you respect your own. Approach them with enlightened love—love that is accepting of what is, without judgment, and with good boundaries.

For my client Roberto, there wasn't anyone he cared less to have a relationship with than his younger brother, Victor. In Roberto's eyes, Victor had "stolen" his life and gotten everything that should have been his. In Roberto's mind, Victor had never had to work for anything—unlike himself. Roberto had grown up on his family farm but had no interest in farming. He dreamed of becoming a lawyer or financier, and worked very hard in school to make his dream a reality. When Roberto was admitted to a prestigious university, he became the first person in his family to go to college. Midway through Roberto's first year away at university, Victor was in a devastating car accident. He was put in an induced coma, and his care team prepped Roberto's parents for the fact that if Victor survived, he'd likely be permanently disabled. Taking care of Victor, who was 14 at the time, became their full-time job. They begged Roberto to take a leave of absence from school and come help them with the farm so that they wouldn't lose their only source of income (and security). Roberto's leave turned into one year, then two, then three. Eventually, Roberto had to terminate his enrollment entirely—the school wouldn't hold his spot for him any longer.

Roberto ended up running the family farm full-time. He expanded his parents' holdings, buying land from surrounding farms and diversifying their crops. He went back to the local agricultural university part-time to further develop his skills and management strategy. The farm became very successful and generated more money than it ever had under Roberto's parents' care. But Roberto still hated farming. He felt trapped, both because it seemed too late to change gears and because his parents relied on him—they could no longer run the farm even if they wanted to; the business of it was now far more sophisticated than it had been during their tenure running it. Meanwhile, Victor had recovered slowly over many years. Though he was permanently disabled physically, cognitively he had no issues. Like Roberto, he was intelligent and driven. And running the farm was definitely out of the question for him—it was too labor-intensive. Victor ended up attending university, the same prestigious one to which Roberto had been admitted and gone for only one semester. It was Victor who went to law school and Victor who became an attorney.

The two brothers hated each other. When I asked Roberto if he knew why Victor hated him, Roberto admitted that it was because his younger brother felt betrayed and hurt by Roberto's anger. Victor thought Roberto was an asshole, pretty much. Roberto knew intellectually that Victor had suffered, and he also knew that Victor did not set out to take anything away from him. Knowing those things didn't change how Roberto felt, though. When Roberto's parents died unexpectedly within a short time of each other, however, Roberto found himself at a crossroads. They had left the farm to him. Roberto wept as he told me he wanted to sell the farm. He was overcome with guilt and with grief.

Roberto and I decided to work on a constellation around the issue of the farm. It became clear that the farm itself was a stand-in for his parents, for his relationship to his parents. By caring for the farm, Roberto had secured their love. He resented Victor not for stealing his life but for stealing that love. Deep down, Roberto never felt as loved by his parents after Victor's accident. Roberto knew that he wanted to sell the farm, but he couldn't without first healing his relationship not only with his parents but also with his brother. The truth is, Roberto never reached a place where he wanted to reconnect with Victor in everyday life—and that's okay. He did make peace with Victor within himself. He worked on letting go of his resentment toward his brother and established better boundaries around "keeping up" with him. He stopped checking Victor's social media and stopped comparing their lives. He acknowledged to himself Victor's own very real and very difficult fate. He accepted the love his parents had had to offer, especially in the form of the farm itself, which was now poised to set him up for life, or close to it. Finally, Roberto sold the farm. In doing so, he became quite wealthy at just 37 years old, and he decided to go back to school and finish his bachelor's degree. At 40, he was accepted to law school. The last time I heard from Roberto, he was pulling all-nighters studying for exams and had never been happier. "Marine, I think I might not actually have liked law school in my twenties," he told me, laughing. "All the years running the farm have really made me deeply appreciate an air-conditioned library. I guess this is the way it was meant to be, because it is the only way it was, you know?"

AFFIRMATIONS

I know my place; my place is my own.

No one else can take or fill my place.

I am secure in who I am and where I belong.

EXERCISE: Belonging Meditation

This meditation is designed to help you deeply embody the principle that everyone has a right place in their family system. I suggest you read it through first, and if you're comfortable doing so, use your smartphone or other device to record yourself reading the meditation. That way, you can listen to the meditation and focus on your visualizations without having to interrupt yourself to check the page for what comes next.

Find a comfortable spot, a space where you can feel peaceful and at ease. You may sit cross-legged or, if you are seated on a sofa or chair, ground your feet on the floor. Allow your palms to rest facing up on your thighs—this is a posture of openness and receptivity, rather than guardedness.

Take three deep breaths and close your eyes. Wherever you are, in this moment, you are safe, you are protected, and you are supported.

At first, all you need to do is connect with your body. Bring your awareness to your body. Feel your feet grounding on the floor; feel your breath in your legs, your hips, your belly, your chest, your arms, your neck, your face. You are completely connected and aligned with yourself. Notice any tension or sensations in your body. Do not try to understand them; just notice them, welcome them.

Now visualize your family. Maybe you see only one person for now; maybe you see 10 or 20. Maybe it's only your parents and your siblings. Or maybe your grandparents are there too; it does not matter. Just ask your family to join you. As they do, do not place them. Just let them come to you and take whatever place they may. Pay attention to any sensations in your body: Do you welcome them? Do you shut them down? Do you want to take some distance; do you want to hide; do you want to run away? Do you want to merge with them? Just bring your attention to where you're drawn to place yourself. Is it near your mother? A sibling? Maybe you want to be in the back. Maybe you want to be in front.

Focus on how it feels to be with your family. Look at them, take them in—all the family members that you called on to join you. And with each of them, you're going to look at them and say out loud or silently, *As you belong, I belong. As you belong, I belong.* Take your time.

Now invite your inner child to join you. The little boy or little girl that you used to be. And again, as with your family, let them find their place. Don't try to control it. Maybe right now your inner child is going to be a bit farther from you, or closer to you, or behind you. Just look at her, look at him, with love, with compassion, and when you feel connected with them, say out loud or silently, *I see you. I hear you. I recognize you. You have a place. And no one can take that place away from you. You have the right to take your place today. And if you don't feel ready yet, that's okay. I will be here for you. I will be standing right here, and I will be waiting for you. I see you, I hear you, and I recognize you. You are important.*

Finally, invite your chosen family—your partner, your children if you have them, your close friends. And again, let them place themselves. You don't need to control them. Just surrender to how, right now, everybody and everything in your life is connected. Look at each person in your chosen family and say, out loud or silently, *It is thanks to my family that I was able to create my chosen family. None of you are here to take care of my past, my healing, my priorities, my responsibilities. We are here to enjoy our life together. So thank you so much. As I honor my past, as I make peace with my childhood, my inner child, I fully welcome my present life, my chosen family. My foundation is my strength. I am in charge of spreading my wings, whenever I want. I can always go back to my family. I belong. I have a place.*

When you feel ready, very slowly and gently open your eyes.

CHAPTER 5

Yes, Yes, Yes

Daddy Issues

We all want to love and be loved. At every turn our culture bombards us in song and story with the message that romantic love is the zenith of fulfillment. And yet, despite our desire and despite our efforts, very few of us seem readily able to enter into or sustain healthy relationships. Six out of every ten people I work with come to me looking to transform their love lives. Either they're struggling in a relationship or struggling to find a relationship, and they're ready for radical change. Most of these people begin either by enumerating everything that's wrong with their partner or reciting a litany of things that are wrong with themselves. A few reference, half-ironically, that old pop-psychology favorite: *daddy issues*. But with almost all of my clients, the problem doesn't actually lie with their partner, with them, or even with the relationship itself—but in unresolved family system issues and the unconscious loyalties, entanglements, and dynamics they produce. Love and relationships are always the natural extension of the dynamics in our family system, and of our inner child's continued quest to demonstrate their loyalty and secure their belonging.

If you took a quick look at my life, there'd be no question about it, right? *Daddy issues*. And like most of my clients, I used to accept the "truth" of it as obvious. But Family Constellations shows us that the truth is often anything but obvious. Like so many of my own clients, I thought the problem with my love life was a simple matter of repetition: I was choosing painful relationships with men because of the hurt I'd experienced with my dad. What I would come to discover instead was the blind love of my inner child, carefully demonstrating her loyalty and securing her belonging.

The strangest day of my life was an otherwise ordinary Sunday in January 2008. It was a chilly but bright Parisian winter day, made colder by dampness and the slush melting on the sidewalks. My brother was home for the weekend from boarding school in Brittany. And the four of us, my mom, my dad, me, my brother, were sitting down for lunch, a ritual we had shared countless times over 20 years. But this would be the last meal we would share as a family for more than a decade.

Over the previous weeks, my mom and I had packed box after box in preparation for our move to the new apartment we'd be sharing. As we'd wrapped our dishes in newspaper and folded our linens, as we'd layered photo albums and books neatly in stacks, as we'd sorted through the accumulated memorabilia of a lifetime, culling the keepers from the giveaway pile, we'd never even mentioned what was happening. After 28 years of marriage, my parents were divorcing.

It had been a year since it became clear that *something* was amiss between my parents—my mom had been increasingly absent, traveling for work incessantly (from my perspective, her coping mechanism for managing pain and worry), and my relationship with my father, never the easiest since I'd become a teenager, grew even stonier and more silent as we moved around each other in our house, avoiding contact. Still, they never told us directly what was happening; my brother and I were left to piece things together from context clues. My parents had always kept any difficulties in their marriage private: They never fought in front of us and they always presented a united front, something I had always been grateful for. But now . . . it was a bit like I was going crazy. Nothing was normal, nothing would ever be normal again, yet we were all pretending as if it were. *Nothing to see here.*

It took only a moment for that illusion to finally become completely unsustainable, though. I remember looking up at the kitchen clock, wondering how much more time we had before my brother needed to leave to catch his train, when my father began to speak. His tone was formal bordering on indifferent. "Listen, I have no animosity toward you," he said. He was speaking *to me and my brother*. "But if your mom leaves, we won't be a family anymore. It's either the four of us, or it's over."

I don't remember the rest of the afternoon. I know my brother tried to speak with him, to reason with him, to insist that *just because you and Mom are divorcing doesn't mean we need to stop seeing each other*. That went nowhere, the only evidence of the conversation the damaged mailbox that had absorbed my brother's fury on his way out of our home. The next morning, my father got up very early and left for work before my mother and I were awake so he would not have to see us leaving the house. We did not say good-bye. That Sunday lunch was the last time I saw my father for the remainder of my twenties.

For seven years, my father refused to speak to or have any contact with us. My brother saw him once in that time, when my father entered the salon where he was having his hair cut—my father, spotting him, just turned and left, refusing to acknowledge him. The only exception to this came a few years into his silence, after I'd had a dream that my paternal grandmother had died. With no small amount of hesitation, I e-mailed my dad, asking after my grandmother. I ended the note, "I hope you are well." My father's scathing reply went something like, "Your grandmother is alive. As for me, how could I be well? Your mother left me. I am alone." *You are alone?!* I couldn't believe he saw himself as the victim or expected *me* to be sorry for *him*. You *are alone?! You cut your own children out of your life.*

By August 2008, just eight months after my dad stopped speaking to me, I was married to a man I'd known only two months. The relationship, initially intoxicating, rapidly turned toxic—controlling and abusive. Within a year we were separated and then divorced, though we dallied with each other, painfully, for several years after that. In 2014, I married a second time and again, it didn't work out. Two failed marriages under my belt by 30. And with every relationship between and since, I have found a way, consciously or unconsciously, to sabotage my chance at happiness, despite how much I want love.

As an adult, whatever is left unresolved in your family system you will re-create in a romantic relationship. Fear of intimacy, fear of commitment, putting up walls, neediness, lack of trust, jealousy, infidelity, loss, self-sabotage—whatever you were unable to heal in your family dynamics, whatever you could not make sense of, whatever you could not solve, there is a 90 percent chance you will "ask" your partner to take care of it for you. I don't mean you will explicitly request something of your partner, but that through the dynamic with your partner you will seek to subconsciously heal old wounds. Your partner will be your next target. The uncomfortable truth is that there is no coincidence in love; you don't choose your partner randomly.

Yes, conventional wisdom has it that we choose partners who remind us of our parents (applied to hetero folks, typically your opposite-sex parent). But this isn't what I'm getting at here. Like most conventional wisdom, it's a little bit right but mostly a lot wrong. Most of my clients, most of us, do not choose partners who *overtly* remind us of our mother or father (in fact, I think for most of us, there'd be a big *ick* factor in doing so). And most of us don't overtly seek to replay history. We don't think, *Oh, my grandmother was widowed before she was 50 and so was my mom, so let me find a partner who will die young.* When we use relationships to resolve family system issues, it's less about the type of person our parents were and more about the dynamics between us or the larger dynamics in the system—and how they shape our current relationships.

One of my clients, Lila, had a husband and a father who could not be more different: Her father was introverted, liked to work with his hands, held a series of odd jobs rather than pursue a career, and when angry, withheld affection, subjecting his daughter to the silent treatment; her husband was charismatic and extroverted, a poet, and a tenured professor at a prestigious university who was a champion yeller and hurler of insults when they disagreed. When we started working together, she had become deeply unhappy with the way her life felt limited by what she perceived as her husband's overwhelming negativity; it seemed like everything in their life was oriented around something her husband had said no to, as she put it: He didn't want children; he didn't like pets; he was a vegetarian and expected her not to eat meat at home; he didn't like "clutter" and hated to see any of her craft projects out (she was an accomplished knitter and quilter); he didn't want her to have houseplants because he considered them messy. The list went on, from the petty and mundane to the life-altering.

Lila described a tense childhood with her father, who angered easily (though quietly) and took any request—for his time, for his attention, for a trip to a park, for a toy or a treat—as a personal affront. "I knew just asking him for something would annoy him," she told me. "If we went somewhere like the park and an ice cream truck pulled up, I wouldn't even bother asking him if we could get something. I knew asking him would annoy him and his answer would be no anyway." As she spoke the last sentence, she faltered. It was the first time she had ever articulated out loud the central theme of her dynamic with her dad: *no*. For the 14 years she had known her husband, she had always remarked how different he was from her father—but all along, she had been reenacting the same dynamic, one in which she subsumed and denied her needs to keep the peace.

Why she was repeating this dynamic is of course the heart of the matter: When it comes to unresolved family system issues and our relationships, it's so often a matter of our inner child still trying to prove their loyalty and earn their belonging. In Lila's case, she never felt heard by her father; he wasn't available to her or to meet her needs. When children don't feel heard, they don't feel they belong. They feel rejected. In continuing this dynamic with her husband, Lila's inner child was still trying to demonstrate to her father that she was a good girl who did, indeed, belong. That was how she knew to demonstrate love and loyalty: acquiescing, even when—especially when—it meant sacrificing her own hopes and dreams.

In the years of silence that elapsed between my dad and me, I would get occasional reports on him from family friends and acquaintances. One of my best friends still lived in the Parisian suburb where I'd grown up, and where my dad was still residing, in what had been our family home. Every time we spoke, she would update me on the seeming absence of life at the house. "Marine," she would tell me, "the shutters are always drawn. It looks like no one lives there." "Marine, the house looks abandoned." When my dad and I saw each other again for the first time in 2015, I was surprised by how different he seemed—it was like the spark had gone out of him. I thought about the lifeless house he had been haunting for the better part of the last decade, how he was moving like a ghost through his own life. Even now, though he has reconnected with my brother and me, an act of love and thus of life, I believe the divorce remains heartbreaking for him.

And all along, I have been loyal to him, deeply so, despite—or because of—his abandonment. When my dad left, when he essentially disowned me, a fundamental part of my identity was severed: my identity as my father's daughter. I lost my sense of self and have been trying to recover it ever since. When my dad left, when he rejected his place in my family system, he created a tear in its fabric that I've been trying to repair ever since. Not through "replacing" his love via my ill-fated marriages, but through loyalty to his own heartbreak. For the last 12 years, I've worked, without realizing it, to prove to my father that I do belong to him. If his heart was broken, so will be mine.

We always remain loyal to our families, especially to our parents. The fierce, blind love of our inner child burns in each of us, regardless of whether we consciously sense it, whether we are aware of it, whether we repudiate our family or embrace it. We will do what we must to right the wrongs of our family system, even as we get it wrong, even as we harm ourselves. We will do what it takes to restore belonging, our own or others'. Of course, the unresolved issues each of us carries from our family systems are too particular, too individual, too diverse and plentiful to even try to list them comprehensively—but that's not my goal. Rather than attempt to iterate all the ways that our parents could have fucked up, or all the ways that a family system can go haywire, I want you to remember the primary duty of a parent (beyond passing on the gift of life): guaranteeing a child's belonging through making sure that they are **seen**, that they are **heard**, that they are **recognized**.

The adult dynamics that undermine connection or prevent us from entering into relationships—fear of intimacy, fear of commitment, putting up walls, neediness, lack of trust, jealousy, infidelity, loss, refusal to grow up, etc.—are almost always an expression of a failure to be seen, heard, or recognized by a parent in childhood: violations of precedence and priority, taking the place of a parent's partner, taking care of our parent's feelings, merging with a parent, rejecting a parent, experiencing a break in a bond, being subject to abuse, etc. It's no surprise to me that most of my clients who come in to work on romantic relationship issues describe their problems *with their partners* in just those terms. I hear more times than I can count: "I don't feel seen," "My partner doesn't listen to me," "I feel rejected."

I had a client who became her parents' go-between after their divorce. They could not speak with each other or be civil toward each other. Suddenly, at age five, my client had to become the grown-up in the relationship, acting as a bridge between her parents. She wasn't *seen* for who she was—a child, their child. Now, in her adult relationship, she wants to be the child, expecting her husband to baby her and take on the majority of the emotional labor between them.

Another client who was perpetually single and unhappy about it described growing up being the caretaker for her father, who had multiple sclerosis. My client was single because, in a sense, she was already in a relationship. She wasn't available—she was her dad's partner; her inner child felt guilty betraying him by moving on with her own life.

With the oldest children in large families, there is often a dynamic in which that child becomes a substitute parent for their younger siblings, charged with endless diaper changing, feeding, babysitting. With their partner, they may feel a sense of "Don't you dare ask me to do anything that I don't want to." The sub-text is "Because I was responsible at a very young age, I refuse to be even more responsible now." They may refuse to take on any mutual responsibility with their partner—paying bills, arranging for home repairs, doing the grocery shopping, cooking, laundry, etc.—causing great strain between them.

As adults, children who have had to stop school or couldn't go to school in order to work to help support their families often transfer their resentment to their partners, often in the form of cheating or financial infidelity. There is a feeling of "I didn't get to have the life of my choosing, so I'm entitled to do what I want now."

An unresolved dynamic with a parent may condition how you *respond* to your partner. Let's say you didn't feel heard by your father growing up. And one evening, your partner isn't paying attention to what you're saying. They're tired; they've had a long day at work. But to you, this may feel at a subconscious level like the rejection you experienced as a child. You explode at your part-ner as a result: "You never listen to me!" To your partner, this outburst will probably seem bizarre and disproportionate to the situation at hand, possibly hurtful or even exhausting if this is a fight you've had before. In this scenario, you're not even upset with your partner, really. It's the little girl or little boy inside of you lashing out, transferring to your partner the hurt and anger he or she feels toward your father. You're transferring the respon-sibility of the past onto the present, demanding that your partner compensate for your parent or that they stand in for the parent who let you down.

My client Anne's husband, René, was the youngest of three boys. While he was growing up, his parents always "joked" that they'd been trying for a girl. They'd even had a girl's name picked out. Can you guess what it was? Yes, my friends, it was Renée. Sure, it's a unisex name in France but for the spelling, but still, they named him the same thing they had planned on naming their hoped-for daughter. In a sense, he didn't even get his own name. René grew up feeling that his parents, no matter what they said, really were disappointed that he—and not the little girl they'd been dreaming of—had been born. That he was not enough for them.

René's first great love had broken his heart by telling him she realized she'd never been in love with him. When I met Anne, she was in a bad place in their marriage. She had had an abortion, against René's will and without telling him. They had a son already and following the son, they'd had a miscarriage. After discussing trying again, they decided together they were "one and done." When Anne unexpectedly became pregnant, she told René she did not want another child. They fought bitterly about it, until Anne took the matter into her own hands.

So again, René felt rejected by someone who was supposed to love him. He literally told Anne, "It's like by refusing my sperm you're rejecting me, the person I am."

Since the abortion, René had become hypercritical of Anne's parenting. She also felt that he was alienating her from their son. Every time she wanted to have quality time with their son, René interrupted the moment. "You should do this. You should do that. Oh, you're playing guitar together? Let me show you how. I'll take him to his music lesson." Slowly but surely, he was pushing Anne away, ensuring their son would be madly in love with Daddy. *Daddy knows everything.* And the son can't reject him, won't reject him, of course.

Anne and I discussed how there was a dual dynamic happening: René was, on the one hand, trying to repair his childhood injury through his own child. And on the other hand, he was reliving his childhood dynamic through his wife: doing everything possible so that his partner would reject him, confirming that he was unlovable, confirming that his parents were right.

Of course, unresolved family system issues are not only limited to dynamics with our parents. Entanglements and patterns that repeat over generations in our families can also play out in our relationships. One of my clients had been with his girlfriend for 10 years. He loved her deeply and couldn't imagine spending his life with anyone else. He was ready to buy a home with her and start trying for a family. But despite that, he wasn't "ready" to get married. This had become such a point of contention between them that his girlfriend was seriously ready to leave him. My client was not opposed to marriage in theory; he didn't subscribe to the "It's just a piece of paper" cliché and he clearly wasn't afraid of being "tied down." But every time he thought of proposing, he experienced overwhelming anxiety. As it turned out, in the three prior generations in his family, every first marriage had ended in divorce, followed by a happy second or even third marriage. A constellation revealed his real fear: that by marrying his girlfriend (a marriage that would be his first), he would somehow ruin their relationship and it would inevitably fail. He was so resistant to marriage because he was actually afraid of losing her, not of committing to her.

Another client was at an impasse with her partner regarding having children. She was 35 and her partner, whom she had been with for seven years, was concerned about their remaining window for pregnancy. Though she and her partner were professionally and financially secure enough to raise kids without undue struggle, she felt certain that once they had children, "something" would happen and they wouldn't be able to take care of them. She also worried that her *partner* would regret it and leave her, despite the fact that it was her partner who was pushing for a child. My client came from a line of single mothers: my client's mother had been a teenager when my client was born; my client's grandfather had left her grandmother for another woman shortly after the birth of their daughter (my client's mother); my client's great-grandmother had been widowed with three kids in her twenties. Despite the fact that my client was in her late thirties and was in a happy and solid partnership with the means to care for children, she was entangled in the fates of the women who had come before her.

When we think about our own relationships and how they might be informed or even shaped by past dynamics that long predate them, we can always start by asking: *Do I feel seen? Do I feel heard? Do I feel recognized?* If the answer to any of these questions is no, take the time to really explore why. Give yourself the space to write out your thoughts. Once you've done that, ask yourself if that was the case in your childhood, even if for different reasons. In other words, if you don't feel recognized by your partner (valued for who you are, right now, exactly as you are), ask yourself if you felt recognized in your childhood. Maybe your partner expresses no interest in your work, which feels central to your identity. Perhaps in childhood or adolescence, your parents rejected your gender expression or enforced certain gender roles that felt unnatural to you. Though the two experiences differ in detail, they are both emblematic of a failure to be recognized.

You can also reverse engineer the above by asking yourself, *What are my complaints about my partner? About my relationship?* The answers to these questions can often give us insight into unresolved family dynamics. If your greatest complaint about your partner is that they're emotionally unavailable, for example, you don't feel heard. What does feeling heard look like to you? Given that, did you feel heard in childhood? Think about how you described your parents earlier. Again, the language you use can offer clues to your issues with them. Do you describe your mother as distant? Critical? Depressed after her divorce? Now, does the way you described your relationship or your partner reflect at all how you described your parents and your relationship with them? What are your biggest fears in your relationship? How do they reflect your dynamics with your parents?

Embarking on the path toward illuminating the connections between your family system dynamics and your relationship can be surprisingly healing. When we return an element of control to our actions and behavior and stop acting at the whims and mercy of a disordered family system, we begin the process of positive change. We can see what we're dealing with and make informed choices that are aligned with the highest good of our relationship, rather than in service to our family system. We empower ourselves to reject narratives we didn't author and to write stories that better reflect reality—to say yes to our relationships.

AFFIRMATIONS

My relationship with my partner is not a
vehicle to heal my relationship with my parents.

My loyalty is to the present, not the past.

I say yes to a relationship that faces forward, not backward.

EXERCISE:

A Relationship Inventory—Taking Stock of Relational Dynamics

In this exercise, we dive more deeply and more explicitly into taking stock of how our relationships might be informed or even shaped by past dynamics. You'll want to write your answers down. Let yourself go as in-depth or get as detailed as you'd like. I find sometimes that once you start writing, it can be surprising how much you suddenly have to say.

Start with your current relationship. If you are single, skip the first set of questions. For the second set of questions, which regard past relationships, complete a set for every relationship you feel has been significant to you, regardless of duration. Only you know which relationships have truly been impactful—even a month-long fling can potentially teach us a lot about who we are and what we want.

Current relationship:

- When you started this relationship, what were your expectations of it?

- When you started this relationship, what were your expectations of your partner?

- Do you feel seen by your partner? If not, why?

- Do you feel heard by your partner? If not, why?

- Do you feel recognized by your partner? If not, why?

- What do you feel is most difficult in this relationship? In other words, what are the greatest sources of conflict that arise between the two of you?

- What do you feel is most lacking? In other words, what do you feel is missing between the two of you?

- Do you repeatedly blame your partner for certain issues? If yes, what are they?

- Do you repeatedly criticize your partner for certain behaviors, actions, or traits? If yes, what are they?

- Finally, be completely honest and try your best to set aside any defensiveness you may feel: What would your partner say is most lacking in this relationship?

Prior relationships:

- When you started the relationship, what were your expectations of it?

- When you started the relationship, what were your expectations of your partner?

- Did you feel seen by your partner? If not, why?

- Did you feel heard by your partner? If not, why?

- Did you feel recognized by your partner? If not, why?

- What was most difficult in the relationship? In other words, what were the greatest sources of conflict that arose between the two of you?

- What did you feel was most lacking? In other words, what did you feel was missing between the two of you?

- Did you repeatedly blame your partner for certain issues? If yes, what were they?

- Did you repeatedly criticize your partner for certain behaviors, actions, or traits? If yes, what were they?

- Did you end the relationship? If so, what was your reason for doing so?

- Did your partner end the relationship? If so, what was his or her reason for doing so?

Now that you've answered these questions for all the relationships you've deemed important to your personal history, take the time to compare your answers for each relationship. Do any patterns emerge? When and how did you answer similarly? Make a list of all of your overlapping answers (e.g., "Didn't feel seen—John, Alex, and Mark").

Next, we'll look at the dynamics with your parent or parents. Complete the set for each parent separately. I use "mother/father" here, but if you grew up with same-sex parents, of course please answer a set of questions for each. If you had a relationship with only one parent, answer only regarding that parent. If you grew up with parent figures or legal guardians (such as grandparents), answer in relation to them. Several of the questions speak to both the past and the present. When it comes to our parents, old habits can be hard to break.

Relationship with parent:

- Growing up, did you feel seen by your mother/father? If not, why?

- Growing up, did you feel heard by your mother/father? If not, why?

- Growing up, did you feel recognized by your mother/father? If not, why?

- What is and/or was most difficult in the relationship? In other words, what were the greatest sources of conflict that arose between the two of you?

- What is and/or was most lacking? In other words, what did you feel was missing between the two of you?

- Did/do you repeatedly blame your mother/father for certain issues? If yes, what were/are they?

- Did/do you repeatedly criticize your mother/father for certain behaviors, actions, or traits? If yes, what were/are they?

Do you see any of the patterns that emerged across relationships in your answers about your parents? Which ones? Write them down. Is there any overlap between individual answers about a partner and answers about your parents? Which ones? Write them down.

Now that you've mapped the potential overlap of patterns in your adult relationships with your parental dynamics, ask yourself for each overlap: *Is this really about my partner, or am I projecting on them past issues with my parents that have remained unresolved?* If the issues with your partner are real, ask yourself, *Am I choosing this partner in order to heal my past?* As tough as this is, ask yourself, *Does this relationship really serve my highest good?* Ask yourself, *If I set aside my attempt to heal my past through this relationship, is what is left enough for me to commit to? Is there the possibility for enlightened love between my partner and me?*

Staying in a relationship or deciding to end it is an extremely personal choice. But making either decision from a place of enlightened love, and then doing the work to follow through from that place, isn't possible without starting with self-awareness. No matter what, saying yes to relationships begins, as ever, with a fearless recognition of reality as it is, not as we wish it to be.

Say Yes

The foundation of a good relationship requires more than just awareness and resolution of unresolved family system issues, though. Yes, doing so enables us to show up for our relationships right here, right now, without subjecting them to the burdens of the past. But once we're here, unburdened, what do we do? We say yes.

Saying yes is hard. Saying yes is consenting to reality. Saying yes means engaging in enlightened love. Saying yes does not mean approval or endorsement—but it can feel that way, causing us to resist. When we say yes, we are saying, "Yes, this is real life. I can control myself, but I cannot control another person."

A good relationship requires that we say yes three times. First, you must say yes to your partner exactly as he or she is, without wanting to change them. This means saying, with 100 percent authenticity, "I say yes to you." It means saying yes to your partner's past: their past partners, their experience of their sexuality, their mistakes, their history. Our partners are not projects; they are not fixer-uppers. We can hope they will change and grow as they experience life, just as we would hope for ourselves, but that is different than hoping they will change in a specific way that you find more pleasing, more palatable, or better suited to your vision of your future. If your partner has spent their twenties rootless, tells you they love to travel and that they do not foresee ever wanting children, you cannot decide that you will change their mind and they'll settle down after marriage. If your partner has never left their hometown and tells you they want to stay close to their family, you cannot decide that you will persuade them to move across the country to the city you prefer. If your partner is unambitious, too ambitious, a workaholic, emotionally avoidant, needy, allergic to cats, messy, a clean freak, whatever—this is who they are. They may choose to go to therapy or alter their lifestyle or have an epiphany, but this is not something you get to initiate, control, or count on.

Second, you must say yes to your partner's family, exactly as it is. This one is tricky. It's obviously a problem when your partner is close with their family but you don't like them. How many times have I heard, "Marine, I love my husband, but I hate his family" (there is usually a difficult mother-in-law relationship lurking in there). This is impossible. Your partner is a product of their family system. When you reject the family, you reject your partner. Your partner likely still shares, to some degree, the values and beliefs of their family of origin. If your partner rejects their family, however, this does not mean *you* should reject their family (again, in doing so, you reject your partner). This is where it gets especially tricky, because it is also never your place to try to force your partner to reconcile with their family. This one can be hard for those of us who are close to our families. We think, *But they would be happier if they were at peace with their father,* or *How could someone really not want a close bond with their mother?* We see ourselves as the hero who will fix their story and restore order to their system. But that is not our role. Saying yes to your partner's family exactly as it is means saying yes to your partner's relationship to his or her family.

Third, and finally, you must say yes to your own destiny and to the destiny of your partner. This is easier to do when you have said yes with clear eyes to your partner as they are and to your partner's family as it is. When you have done so, you are grounded in reality. Your vision is unclouded and the path ahead becomes sharper. And sometimes, as painful as it may be, saying yes to your destiny and to your partner's destiny means acknowledging that your paths are diverging. Your destinies are moving away from each other.

I see so many of my clients in pain because they are holding on to a relationship that no longer serves them or their partner. The reasons for doing so are, as ever, deeply individual, but also universal: fear of being alone, the sunk cost fallacy, shared children, inability to withstand conflict, and so on. But when we stay in a relationship that no longer serves our destinies, we stop having agency in our own lives. We perpetuate dysfunctional dynamics and set ourselves up for failure. Sometimes, nurturing a "good" relationship means knowing when to end it, and how: with respect and love.

Remember, I did say that saying yes is hard. Ending a relationship, even a very bad one, with respect and love is a way of saying yes. It does not mean agreeing to the ways in which the relationship was painful or how your partner may have hurt you (or how you may have hurt them). Respect means *respecting your shared story*. It means taking responsibility for your part in your relationship and acknowledging that through that relationship you have arrived where you are now—acknowledging all you have learned, all that you take away from the relationship. When we end a relationship with respect, we accept reality, and we accept what is beyond our power to control: other people.

Love means *enlightened love*. Remember, when love is enlightened, we see people for who they are, without judgment; we are able to acknowledge not only their flaws but also what they have given us. When we end a relationship with love, we don't engage in berating our former partners (or ourselves) or living in our anger perpetually.

The more we reject our former partners, the more we reject ourselves. We reject that earlier version of ourselves, who sought out that love for whatever reason. We reject our vulnerability; we reject our mistakes; we reject our own history and what it has to offer us. It isn't unlike your dynamic with your parents: The more you can accept and respect your parents, the better able you are to accept and respect yourself. With relationships, the more you can respect your past—the more you respect priority, what came first—not only will you be better grounded in the present moment, but you will be better able to choose a partner who respects and accepts you, and better able to accept and respect your next partner.

I have had clients who feel that they treated their former partner with respect and love in ending a relationship, but who still nurse deep-seated anger toward them. Look, this just isn't possible—you can't have ended things with respect and love but still feel red-hot rage about it. You might have gone through the motions of respect and love; your outward behavior may have been spotless. But when we are still deeply angry with a former partner, we are still de facto entangled in that relationship, which means it did not end properly. And when we are still entangled in a previous relationship, there is no way to be truly, 100 percent available to our current partner or open to a next partner. On the other side of the spectrum, I also have clients who claim to feel nothing toward their former partners. This is also bullshit, sorry. We are made of feelings. When we "feel nothing," we are engaging in a coping mechanism to protect ourselves from pain. When you end a relationship with respect and love, you don't feel nothing—you feel at peace. At peace with what was, at peace with your choices, at peace with your partner.

Here's the thing: A relationship might technically end after a breakup, but it may live on within us for quite some time. After all, a relationship is separate from the people who entered it. The relationship is what you created between you. It doesn't just disappear when a person exits your life or take on a new role in your life (as with a co-parent). Ultimately, ending a relationship with respect and love is about ending it *within yourself.* Yes, you should do your best to end things with love and respect in the moment, but none of us can fast-forward our way to peace. You make room for it by allowing yourself to mourn, by accepting what is, and by extending that enlightened love first toward yourself. And remember, your ability to choose respect and love isn't contingent upon your ex-partner's behavior. Many of us have experienced ex-partners who are neither respectful nor loving, who seem to live to make us miserable after we part ways. When that is the case: boundaries, boundaries, boundaries, boundaries. No one else gets to control how you feel.

I see both situations—unresolved anger or an absence of emotion—primarily after relationships that were particularly painful, such as when cheating was involved, or that were, horribly, emotionally or physically abusive. I will never pretend that coming away from a relationship like this with love and respect is easy. It may take a long time to get there. That's okay. I've been there. And it's understandable to say, "Why should I want to?" In the next chapter, we'll dig deep about consenting to reality—saying yes—after trauma.

For now, this is what I want you to hold on to: When you end a relationship with love and respect, as we discussed it, you are saying yes to your destiny—you are choosing yourself. The problem in so many relationships is that we choose our partners instead; we put them first. This is disorder, quite literally. You come first in your own system. Make yourself happy first, and then you can share that happiness with a partner. Instead, what happens 90 percent of the time is something much more transactional—we put our partners first, with the hope that in making them happy, they will make us happy. *I will see you, so you will see me. I'm going to love you, so you will love me.* This is not love. This is co-dependency.

You have to feel secure in your love for yourself first. You have to feel safe with yourself before you ask a partner to make you feel safe. The problem is, when we shift that responsibility to our partner, we alienate ourselves from knowing and understanding our own boundaries. Not to mention we are bound to be disappointed. Our ways of feeling safe and secure in a relationship are likely to be different from our partner's, as we grew up in different homes with different expressions of love. Their way of expressing love may feel foreign to us and thus unsatisfying; the goal is to arrive at a mutual understanding of what the other needs and meet them there. When only one particular expression of love is acceptable, when we demand adherence to our norm rather than open ourselves to what is, the relationship becomes fragile. Our wounded inner child, who wasn't fulfilled by the love their parent had to offer (but which was the only right love for them, as it was the only love there was), has taken the wheel. This is where accepting our parents and saying yes to what is comes back into play: When we have done so, when we work to heal the wounds our inner child has sustained, we learn how to be safe with ourselves. We learn how to create healthy boundaries. We love ourselves first. We choose ourselves first.

If you don't feel safe and secure with yourself, you may disregard the early signs of an abusive relationship. These often reveal themselves quickly, though in small ways at first, which can be easy to miss or acquiesce to. Your partner might insult you: "Wow, you didn't know X? How stupid." How you react hinges on that sense of self. A person who feels secure and safe with themselves might respond, "Listen, maybe you think it was stupid, but I would ask you to respect me," because they have that self-confidence to know that *No, I am not stupid, I just did not understand something.* This is self-love. They are saying to themselves and to their partner, *Hold on a minute here! That's my life. I respect my life. And that's exactly what I ask of you in return: to respect my life.* When we answer instead, "Oh my god, I am so stupid; I'm sorry," we are not choosing ourselves; we are choosing our partner and our partner's "safety" first.

My first husband completely swept me off my feet when I was young, dumb, and vulnerable. Our two-month courtship was a blur of intense sex, declarations of undying passion, and the feeling that someone was madly in love with me, quite literally— there was a madness, an insanity, an unbalanced, unstable nature to my husband's "love," which was more like an obsession. Within months of our impulsive Las Vegas wedding, his controlling, domineering, and jealous behaviors had blossomed into full-fledged violence. Though all the signs were right there at the beginning— red flag after red flag—I was blinded by my much greater need to feel seen and desired, which the relationship provided to a degree I had never experienced before. My self-worth had been utterly crushed under the bootheel of my father's rejection earlier that year. And, to be honest, my father had always been distant, an enigma even as I had lived side by side with him for the previous 22 years. When it came to my new husband, at first I didn't even question his love. I didn't think his behaviors were weird or that I was in danger. I constantly chose him first, so that he would choose me. I wasn't safe or secure with myself.

My husband had his own unresolved issues to contend with, I understand now. He was the middle child of three sons, and his younger brother—whom he loved fiercely—was severely disabled and died at the age of 12. Despite how much he loved his brother, he was also jealous and resentful of him while growing up. He was incredibly angry with his mother, who'd had to devote a large part of her life to caring for his little brother and was then undone by grief when he died. He once told me a story about how he'd had to be hospitalized after an accident in his childhood. While he was sleeping, his mother had to leave the hospital briefly to go back home and care for his little brother. She slipped off the bracelet she always wore and left it, with a note telling him she loved him and she would be back soon, on his bed, so he would see it first thing when he woke up. When he told me this story, I felt so sad for his mother. I thought about how difficult it must have been to leave her son in the hospital, how torn she must have felt, how guilty. But my husband saw it as an unforgivable betrayal, even all those years later. "Who leaves their child alone in a hospital?" he said. "What kind of mother was she?"

Deep down, my husband believed all women would betray him, would leave him, like his mother had. He was a jealous person who wanted to be left so that he could prove he was right in his rejection of his mother—and by extension, all women. A few years after we divorced, he attempted to apologize. "I can see now that you were everything that I was looking for, but I was afraid," he said. "You were not afraid," I answered. "Your little boy was afraid—but the situation was between you and your mother and not between you and me."

I tell you all of this not to excuse my husband—there is no excuse and never will be for what he did—or to imply that you should feel sorry for him. I don't. He is an adult and responsible for his actions. But developing an understanding of what drove us both has helped me to say yes to that relationship. It has removed the shame I felt for staying with him. It has helped me let go of anger, to finally, finally end the relationship with love and respect. Respect for my story and enlightened love for what I took from it. We were two broken people whose unresolved family system issues complemented each other perfectly, perpetuating a cycle of loneliness and rage. Saying yes has helped me to choose myself first going forward, and to feel safe and secure with myself.

Even if you've never been in an abusive relationship, almost all of us have been in relationships that have had issues, from minor to serious. All relationships have issues at times. But regardless of the quality of the relationship, or the nature of our partner, there is a constant: We must say yes to it. At its most basic, this means simply accepting that you did, in fact, choose to enter into the relationship—it didn't just happen to you. We are always responsible for our participation in the relationship. In a relatively "healthy" relationship, this means accepting that you played or play some part in its dysfunctional elements or friction points. In a damaging or toxic relationship, this means acknowledging how the relationship served you initially, even if that is difficult to confront. Doing so does not mean that you deserved the treatment. Doing so does not mean that you approve of what happened to you. Doing so does not excuse the other person's behavior. It simply means that you are acknowledging the full picture so that you are better equipped to choose yourself in the future.

You are responsible for your life. You are not responsible for what happened to you in childhood. But in adulthood you do get to choose, to a large degree, what you want for yourself, including your relationships. You may have lacked self-awareness, you may have been entangled, you may have been unconsciously trying to heal old wounds, but your choices were still your own. However uncomfortable it makes you, it's a truth you must accept. When we avoid the truth of our responsibility for ourselves, we miss out on what our relationships have to teach us about ourselves: what we really need, what we will and won't accept. We miss out on better understanding our motivations—and avoiding self-sabotaging behaviors. You can't learn from your relationship when you insist that you played no part in it. After all, what is there to learn about yourself when you did nothing?

When we avoid the truth of our responsibility for ourselves, we aren't able to say yes to our destiny—to choose ourselves—because we haven't said yes to reality. The more practice we have at choosing ourselves, however, the more safe and secure we feel in ourselves, and the more likely we are to find and sustain the great love we deserve.

AFFIRMATIONS

I say yes to my partner exactly as he or she is.

I say yes to my partner's family exactly as they are.

I say yes to my destiny and to the destiny of
my partner, even if our paths diverge.

EXERCISE: Respecting Your Shared Story

I really hate the phrase "Everything happens for a reason." Bad things happen all the time, without reason, and there is often nothing that can lessen the pain of the bad thing. That said, I do believe that every experience, no matter how painful, offers us the opportunity (at some point) to *learn*: learn about ourselves, about others, about what it means to be human. What we learn shapes us. Relationships are some of the richest sources for this kind of learning. That's why I write that respecting the story of your relationship (a story you share with your relationship partner) means acknowledging that through that relationship you have arrived where you are now, acknowledging all you have learned, all that you take away from the relationship. But where do you start? That's what this exercise is all about: giving you a focused, rather than comprehensive, way to think about what your relationships have to teach you about yourself. It's meant to be a catalyst for a longer, ongoing conversation. I encourage you to approach the exercise from a broad perspective, thinking about the history of your relationships overall, rather than one relationship in particular. After all, how does the saying go? *Meet one asshole today and you've met an asshole. Meet three assholes today and you're the asshole.* Patterns, patterns, patterns—it's the Family Constellations way.

Remember the Relationship Inventory you just did? (Of course you do.) Grab it. Awesome. We are going to use the work you did there and turn it on yourself. As you work through this exercise, take the time to write down your responses without belaboring them. Again, go into as much depth or detail as you'd like or need—you may be surprised at what comes to you once you start writing.

First, I want you to review your answers to the question "When you started the relationship, what were your expectations of it?" Do you see any repeating themes here? What are they? Our expectations for our relationship can reveal to us *what we believe relationships are for*, what purpose they serve: the *why* behind the expectation. Once we've uncovered those beliefs, we can assess whether or not they're actually in alignment with our values.

Look back at your answers to the question "What was most difficult in the relationship? In other words, what were the greatest sources of conflict that arose between the two of you?" Did you experience similar conflicts with more than one partner? What are they? The same conflict repeating with different partners can shine a light on our *own* weak spots, such as in our communication style or in our attachment style.

Next, look over your answers to the question "What did you feel was most lacking? In other words, what did you feel was missing between the two of you?" What we feel is missing in a relationship—physical intimacy, emotional intimacy, romance, etc.—can point us to how we experience love (what feels like love to us, rather than what we tell ourselves love is). If there is a repeating theme here, it can illuminate that we may be on a search for the kind of love we imagine is the real "only right love," the love we feel our parents *should have* given us in childhood.

Practicing facing the less palatable parts of yourself without judgment is an act of bravery and an exercise in saying yes to yourself and your destiny. Taking an opportunity to learn is also taking an opportunity to grow. In acknowledging and accepting any schisms between our beliefs and our actions, we are empowered to close those gaps and be in integrity with ourselves.

CHAPTER 6

From Fragmentation to Wholeness

Survival Instinct

Trauma is a tricky beast. If you experience trauma, you know it informs, even controls, our thoughts, feelings, behaviors—*our very bodies*—without our consent, making itself known when we least expect it. A sight, a sound, a scent, among a million other nuanced and individual triggers, can spark the trauma response, thrusting you out of time as you know it, from the present into the past, a past that feels as alive, terrifying, and inescapable as ever. It's deeply unfair and shitty, to put it mildly, to be forced to relive such fear and pain.

From the Family Constellations perspective, trauma is especially insidious to our well-being not only because of its devastating symptoms but also because of the particular way so many of us attempt to manage those symptoms: through a drive to either erase the past or revisit it (or both, often), which prevents us from living fully in the present or from moving forward into a future of our own choosing—one that is active instead of reactive. In a sense, you could say that living with trauma is like being in an entanglement with yourself.

The drive to erase or revisit the past—to somehow, *somehow*, correct it or fix it—is, in essence, an argument with reality. We know we cannot change the past. Yet we are still, understandably, addicted to our need to try. Are we stuck? NO. Family Constellations tools can help you to gain the critical clarity you need to accurately see yourself in a neutral and nonconfrontational way, as something apart from your trauma. Once you have that tool in your tool kit, you can wield one of Family Constellations' most powerful "secret weapons": *acknowledging what is*—consenting to reality and releasing *yourself* from a toxic victim-perpetrator bond. The healing that results is deep and powerful. I know, because I've been right there with you. When I write *we* and *us* and *our* in these pages, I truly mean it. The rape I experienced at 13 years old locked me in the grip of trauma for 15 years. Family Constellations helped free me from it. And it can liberate you too.

Trauma is, of course, an *extremely* sensitive subject and one that must be handled with great care in any therapeutic setting. Therapists spend years training to specialize in the treatment of trauma. The principles of Family Constellations comprise only one weapon in an arsenal of healing approaches, but I believe it is a powerful one. That said, if you have experienced trauma, I encourage you to seek help from a practitioner trained in working with trauma and to use Family Constellations principles as a complement to your healing work.

When my parents sent me to London at age 13, they did so because they loved me. My trip to London—three weeks in a language immersion program—was meant to secure my future, to open those doors only English-language fluency could unlock. Being bilingual would widen my academic and professional prospects within France; it would mean I could leave France if I wanted; I could study overseas; I could even live and work in the United States one day. The world would be so much *bigger*. That was all my parents wanted for me: opportunity.

They couldn't have known that midway through the program, on a regular afternoon on a random London side street, that an older student would assault me, or that after the rape he would assure me, "You liked that." I had just gotten my period for the first time only a few months earlier; I still played with Barbie dolls.

They couldn't have known that the future they were envisioning for me would be hijacked by the past. They couldn't have known that even as I did move overseas and make a life for myself abroad, my fluency opening all those doors they imagined, I would spend the next 15 years stuck in place, frozen in a gray cobbled alley in London.

And they never would know, because I didn't tell them. Though I was devastated and afraid and confused and wanted my parents to rescue me, or at least to protect me, as any child would, I also wanted to protect my parents—that's the crazy love of children. After all, the assault had taken place on a trip meant as a life-changing gift from them. It was an embodiment of their unconditional love for me. How could I ruin their joy in it? I couldn't. Out of an almost unconscious love and loyalty to my family system, I kept silent.

My sexual assault became my darkest secret, even to myself. I never told anyone about it. In its immediate aftermath, I blacked out. The moments before and after were erased from my memory. How I got back to my host family's home or where Alexandre, my rapist, went, I do not know. All I remember is "coming to" at my host family's home, where I was already on my daily call—6 P.M. sharp—with my parents letting them know that I was fine, even as I floated somewhere above my body. That was the beginning of many years of being outside my body, of a disassociation from my body and my sexuality. In an instant, before I'd even had a chance to discover sex and pleasure and intimacy, I became someone who saw myself as an object, rather than as the owner of my own sexuality. That is one of the hallmarks of trauma: It disassociates us from our bodies, robbing us not only of pleasure in sensuality but of a groundedness, a connection to physicality that is a connection to vitality itself. Take a moment here to check in with your own body. Bring your awareness to your breath and feel it move through you. Flex your toes, your fingers. This is hard and brave and potentially triggering work. Place your feet firmly on the ground. Take another deep breath. Stretch. Honor the beating of your heart.

The inky darkness of the blackout would come to veil the event almost entirely over the following years, until I could and did pretend to be just a regular teenager, then a regular young adult, leading a regular life. I pretended and pretended that I was okay until I just "forgot." I put on a mask and kept living my life compartmentalized, with no connection to the assault. But I wasn't okay. The trauma of the assault had overwhelmed my ability to cope with it, so though I managed to shut it out initially—a classic trauma response—it insisted on making itself known. I had shaking fits regularly. Any time I encountered a mention of rape or sexual abuse, panic would seize my body. My bubble of denial was intermittently punctured by violent and obsessive revenge fantasies that left me ill. My romantic relationships were toxic and abusive. For all of my adolescence and most of my twenties, I wasn't fully living. I was just surviving. It was the best I could do. It's the best so many of us can do in the aftermath of a trauma, isn't it?

As a Family Constellations facilitator, I've met many men and women who are enmeshed in the far-reaching strands of trauma's web. As we know, trauma isn't an event in and of itself but a *response to* an event that has brutally rent one's sense of self and safety (such as war, abuse, rape, accidents, and other forms of violence—be they reoccurring or isolated incidents), overwhelming our ability to cope, stranding us in a feeling of helplessness, and limiting our ability to feel the full array of human emotions. Traumatic events are life-threatening, and our only goal during and in their aftermath is survival.

Our animal instincts equip us with three primary survival strategies: fight, flight, or freeze. You might employ all three strategies at different times, but regardless of whether you are fighting, fleeing, or freezing in the experience, trauma keeps you locked in the embrace of the past. Your life energy becomes dedicated to trying to rewrite what can't be unwritten: The past cannot be undone as much as we may wish it could be. In this way, trauma disconnects you from the natural flow of life, which moves forward in time. With trauma, you circle the past: You may feel compelled to "correct" the trauma and become drawn to situations that resemble the original experience. For example, do you ever find yourself seeking out partnerships that end up repeating themes from a difficult or abusive parent relationship? That would be a corrective strategy. Or you may fixate on a fear of experiencing trauma again and do whatever you can to avoid any setting or situation that is even vaguely similar to the original experience. Think about your own life: Do you ever pass up opportunities that you'd otherwise take because the context even slightly hints at a similarity to your traumatic event? A trip, a job, a social event? That would be the avoidant strategy. (Despite living in New York City and being an EU citizen, I have never returned to London in all these years.) Of course, neither course of action is necessarily that straightforward. The key is to pause and consider the ways in which trauma may have informed your choices and decisions, delimiting the possibilities of your life, even when you were not actively experiencing traumatic symptoms.

Trauma disconnects us from the flow of life because it also has a way of separating us from other people. Just as I never spoke to anyone of my abuse, so many of the men and women I work with treat their traumatic experiences as secrets to be kept at all costs. But when you keep silent, the cost is always to yourself. Even as you attempt to go back to or lead a "regular" life—also a survival instinct to "get back to normal"—your subconscious mind and body refuse to cooperate, refuse to forget. The subconscious mind continues to employ fight, flight, or freeze strategies, and the body manifests the profound stress of living on this kind of high alert. Family Constellations is an integrative modality, so in my practice I am not only listening to my clients' words, but I'm also on the lookout for the physical signs that point to this kind of stress: eyes that constantly scan the room, fists clenched in anger regardless of the subject at hand, the curvature of a back hunched in defensive posture—and I see them every day, while my clients seem not to notice the habits of their own bodies. (Now is a great time for another check-in: What's your posture like? Are your muscles tensed? What are your hands doing? Try to take a moment to actively relax and loosen your body, if you can.)

Sooner or later, the mind and body produce nightmares, flash-backs, and physical symptoms—from tremors to illness—as a way to manage the overwhelm. In these moments, people often turn to alcohol, drugs (legal or illegal), and risky behaviors to self-medicate and numb the pain. However, when the effects of the first dose or drink disappear, the only solution is to double the next intake, and, of course, by doing this we can gradually enter a vicious circle where it is very difficult to get by and lead a full life.

Though not everyone who experiences trauma self-medicates or engages in self-harming behavior, trauma can and does still disrupt life profoundly, over long periods of time, even if you don't attempt to manage its effects in those particular ways. One way of managing might just be shutting down. The simple difficulty of going about day-to-day life while experiencing the effects of trauma can lead to a withdrawal from life and severe anxiety and depression.

Before you dismiss the possibility that you may be depressed, know that depression can manifest in ways that are not always obvious to its sufferers. Because the powerful emotions trauma provokes can be terrifying—I see many clients who learn to be afraid of strong emotion in general, another form of numbing and alienation from the self. In the years after my rape, for example, I became extremely cautious when speaking, since words had been one of my primary vehicles of expressing myself. I had to be in control of them so that I didn't reveal the truth or hurt my family or friends—or myself. Essentially, I silenced my authentic self and was not fully living. It was another act of disassociation that pushed me into a depression I experienced for almost a decade, though it was not always clear to me or others that I was depressed, even as it was happening.

I see this with my clients frequently—people who present as healthy, even as they are in tremendous pain. One of my clients was a 30-year-old fitness instructor and nutritionist who led an Instagram-enviable life of travel and "wellness." Both her parents had died of cancer within a span of 10 years; first her mother when my client was 18, and then her father when she was 28. She had started on her wellness path after the death of her mother. She got interested in yoga and travel, then in more and more restricted diets, and eventually she became a firm adherent of juicing and fasting. On the outside, she looked like a healthy woman, though noticeably thin—but because of her profession her friends and family accepted this as normal, and our culture positively reinforced her appearance as an achievement. Over time, I learned that she was an extreme faster—she fasted every other month for a month at a time. Her extreme skinniness mirrored that of her parents at the ends of their lives. She was slowly willing herself away, following her parents, choosing death, which was disguised as a "healthy" lifestyle. She was simultaneously reenacting the trauma of her parents' illnesses and deaths, even as she attempted to "correct" it through an obsession with diet and exercise—and an ironic disassociation from her body.

Another client I worked with was drawn to relationships that mirrored the dynamic of her trauma, seemingly offering her the possibility of a "redo." She was a very successful designer and in complete control of herself. It took her a few sessions to share her real issue (she had come to me seeking help navigating next steps in her career): Though she was in her mid-thirties, she only dated men in their sixties and seventies. She explained to me that even though they did not typically have sex (due to the simple mechanics of aging and biology), these men treated her "like a princess." In any case, she was not particularly interested in sex or having a family, but she was starting to consider the possibility of dating someone closer to her own age. As we set up her constellation, she revealed that her father had molested her when she was a little girl. In a sense, her relationships with men twice her age allowed her to "correct" that relationship, to reconcile her inner child with her father. Her relationships with older men were transactional, though not in the traditional sense. Instead of trading sex for material goods, she was trading her youth for the sense of being protected and sheltered by an adult—a man old enough to be her father.

In every case, trauma catches us in a closed loop, one in which we are always circling back to the moment of the traumatic event. There's a sense of being condemned to your fate, of stagnation, and of separation from the self and the body, despite the too-often physical manifestations of trauma (which, in fact, only distance you more from being in your body). You're in survival mode. The first step to healing is to actively choose to thrive instead of merely to survive, to choose yourself, to choose the present. Reconnecting with your body is the first seemingly small but actually crucial step in making this choice. When you reconnect with your body, you reject dissociation, and when you push back against dissociation, you begin to exit survival mode. You can teach your body that it no longer has to be on high alert, that it deserves to release that tension, to surrender that burden, to finally relax. To know you are safe. What gives you pleasure? When do you feel most centered in your body? Is it the feel of a freshly laundered cotton T-shirt against your skin? Soaking in a hot spring? The sensation of wind in your hair? Petting a beloved animal? Dripping with sweat during a challenging workout? Eating a piece of the most exquisite chocolate you can find? Walking barefoot in the grass? Whatever it is, stop reading right now and do it—or make an appointment to have it done. Then do it again. Make a commitment to choose yourself, to choose your body, to go beyond survival.

AFFIRMATIONS

I choose life.

I choose recovery.

Healing myself is my priority.

EXERCISE: The Loving Mirror—Choosing Life

Trauma can make it difficult to really see ourselves, wrapped as we are in narratives about what happened to us and mechanisms designed to manage its effects. For this exercise, the goal is small but powerful: to recount the facts of what happened to you with attempted neutrality (i.e., without addressing your feelings about those facts), as you regard yourself lovingly—giving yourself permission to choose to heal. Write down what happened to you and, if you can, look at yourself in the mirror (no obligation) and read what you've written out loud. You will be only with yourself, and you can stop whenever you want. There is no rush. When you stop, connect with your body and your reflection. Rub your arms, feel your pulse, look into your eyes. Take a deep breath and feel the air expanding your chest. You are still here, your heart beating, your body present and real in this moment. You are defiantly alive. To finish, you can repeat the affirmations above. (If it feels safer to do so, this is also an exercise you can try with a therapist, who can function as your "loving mirror.")

Consenting to What Is

In Family Constellations, the goal is not to diminish the enormity of the traumatic event you experienced but to help you disentangle from the hold of the past. When you are liberated from a fixation on the past, you are able to reenter the flow of life— to say *yes* to your own life. The first step to liberating yourself from the past is to *acknowledge what is*. This means to acknowledge what happened to you. When you acknowledge something, you take notice of it. You don't pretend it isn't there. To acknowledge means to hear. Hear your pain, memories, and feelings and in doing so, honor them. Then we *consent to what is*. We accept what happened. This means we accept that what happened, happened, and we can do nothing to alter that reality. *Consenting to what is* is one of the fundamental principles of Family Constellations. But consenting to what is can be especially confusing in relation to trauma, and it is natural to resist doing so. How are you supposed to accept something so awful? Because when you consent to what is, you are *not* agreeing that what happened to you should have happened. Critically, you are also not consenting to your *feelings* about what happened. In other words, you are not agreeing that you are a sad, broken person whose life has been damaged irreparably. Those are your *feelings* about what happened, not facts. You are consenting to *reality* instead of attempting to argue with it. For many of us who experience trauma, we are caught in an argument with reality, insisting, "That should not have happened to me." And of course, it shouldn't have. But it did. So much of the trauma response is about a desire (natural and understandable) to change the past. But the reality is you cannot change the past. You must consent to that reality.

Without consent, your wishes and fears—your constructs—interfere with your perception. When you consent to reality, you recognize simply what is. You focus on the facts, *not on your narratives about those facts*. Not on what could have been or should have been or won't be. You give up trying to find the answer to "Why?" Doing so produces a clarity of perception that is liberating—*What happened to me is not my identity; it is only an experience.*

This is the power and promise of consenting to what is: It liberates you from the stranglehold of the traumatic event because it separates you from your traumatic experience. When you consent to reality, you decenter yourself and depersonalize the event: What happened is not an event *about* you; it is an event that happened *to* you. Yes, it is an experience that informs how you see the world. It is also only one experience among many—a piece of you, but not what defines who you are.

You can practice consenting to *what is* in lower-stakes ways every day, just to build the muscle. Seriously, try it out on someone you know, with whom you have a complicated but not traumatic relationship. This could be a parent, an ex, a friend, a sibling—you get the idea. For our purposes here, you should feel safe doing so. Look at a picture of this person or hold the image of him or her in your mind. Now try saying, "I acknowledge you as my [sister]; I accept you as my [sister]; I consent to what has happened between us." Remember what this process really means: Reality is never wrong, no matter how much that may suck. Here, you're acknowledging that your sister is, indeed, your sister. You are accepting the reality that she is your sister, regardless of how you may feel about this reality. And you are consenting to the reality of what has unfolded or happened in the course of your relationship—agreeing to the fact that it did happen and cannot be undone. There's a kind of *relief* in simply stating the truth without the overlay of narrative, after all the effort you've likely expended in trying to change reality.

I don't minimize the effects of trauma—for 15 years of my life, I struggled with its effects. But when you consent to what is, you engage in an enormous act of respect for yourself. Just as Family Constellations asks us to respect the fate of others in our family systems—even those with difficult destinies—we must respect our own fates.

When we respect our fate, when we acknowledge what is and consent to reality, to the cards we have been dealt through no fault of our own, we are free to forge our own destinies. We become the authors of our own stories. Our various fates are only the building blocks of those stories. How we choose to structure and shape that narrative is up to us. One of my clients is a writer who has taught writing for many years. As we discussed the concepts of consent and fate, she had an epiphany. "Oh," she said, "it's like when I give a class of students a series of writing prompts. They all get the same prompts—the same suggested characters or contexts or situations—but each one writes a different story."

Our futures are unwritten. We are the authors of our lives. When we are locked in mortal combat with the past, we foreclose the possibility of the future. Through consenting to what is, Family Constellations helps to diminish the hold of the past on our present. It does not diminish the event, but it helps to heal its effects by diminishing its ongoing power and restoring it to the larger context of our lives, rather than treating it as the context in which the rest of our lives unfold.

Trauma is a fact of life. It does not have to be a life sentence, however. While you will never forget your trauma—nor should you—you are more than a reflection of your circumstances. Happiness is an achievement of the soul. For my part, consenting to what is helped me to make a radical peace with that piece of my story. The clarity of perception I achieved illuminated a new reality—or perhaps, better stated, it allowed me to see the reality that had always been there: My trauma does not define me. I am the one who defines me. Accepting the reality of the past without judgment released me from its spell and freed me to tell a new story.

Your trauma does not define you. You are the one who defines you. Stop fighting reality; stop battling the trauma. You won't "win." It won't go anywhere. Surrender to what is. Release it with love and acceptance, and finally reinclude this episode in its place in the past, where it belongs. Let's free ourselves from fear, shame, guilt, and anger. Let us see ourselves accurately: as individuals empowered with agency, who continue moving forward despite—or even because of—the obstacles we encounter on the path of our destiny.

AFFIRMATIONS

I will no longer argue with reality; I consent to what is.

My trauma does not define me. I am the one who defines me.

I am not broken; I love myself more than I did before.

EXERCISE:

New Perspectives, New Stories—Reframing Your Narratives

This exercise is inspired by my client who taught writing and her observation that given the same set of prompts, her students would each tell a different story, each filtered through the lens of their particular relationship to the world: their cultures, education, and experiences, among many influences coming together to shape the unique stories they told from the same raw material. In other words, their stories were dependent on their perspectives.

The traumatic event is only one of the factors among many in your own life that has informed your perspective: how you see yourself, how you understand the direction of your life, and how that mediates your relationship to the world around you. We cannot rewrite the traumatic event—that would be arguing with reality. But we *can* build the skill of surrendering our old narratives and writing new and different narratives around how we see ourselves and how we understand the direction of our lives, even with the same set of preconditions. The skill lies in the interpretation of those preconditions—of shifting negative perception to positive perception. We can learn how to see through a different lens; we can change our perspective. This skill is valuable not only in integrating and accepting traumatic events but also in reframing many kinds of experiences—such as personal, professional, and academic failures *and* successes—as sources of personal development that increase our clarity about what we need, deepen our self-knowledge, and serve our growth.

This exercise is meant to be a gentle way to practice perspective shifting. It's all about building the *skill* itself. So, to build those muscles for the heavy lifting of trauma-related work, we'll start with a lower-stakes example from your current life. Divide a sheet of paper into three columns. Think about a concrete issue in your daily life that's frustrating you. Now label the first column "The Issue," the second column "Perspective," and the third column "Alternates."

In the first column, identify your issue briefly and in a fact-based manner. Example: "I have a prestigious job that pays well, but I am no longer engaged or fulfilled by the work." In the second column, express your current perspective on the situation, keeping the focus on your feelings (this isn't about other people). Example: "I'm too old/have invested too much time building this career to switch career paths now." In the third column, list three alternative perspectives (it can be helpful to enlist a friend or family member here) on the situation. Example: "1. This is an opportunity to explore whether I'm really unhappy in this career or in this *particular* job. 2. Time will pass no matter what, and in two to three years I will be older regardless, and potentially still unhappy. I might as well go back to school/learn a new skill/do job training. 3. My attachment to my job is about its *prestige*—about outside approval—and does not stem from my inner, personal values."

Now choose one of the alternative perspectives. Practice holding it close at mind—almost like a mantra—for the next three days. You can meditate on the alternate perspective for a minute at a time when you wake up or before you go to sleep, and throughout the day when the issue arises. At the end of the three days, check in with yourself. How has your perspective shifted? What lesson has emerged? Is there a different story to be told about your current situation?

Releasing Blame

I'm going to go out on a limb here and guess that you've been told or have heard that forgiveness is one of the keys to healing your trauma. There are many takes on what constitutes forgiveness, but broadly, I think it's fair to say that therapeutic culture upholds forgiveness not only as an act you perform for someone else but also (and more importantly) as a service you do for yourself, a way of releasing anger and moving on with your life. With forgiveness, the theory goes, you let go of your hold on the past—on what happened—and are freed from focusing on the one who harmed you, so that you can devote your attention to the present. On the surface, it doesn't seem *so* different from consenting to what is, right?

I heard the same thing too. Many times, on the path toward healing—before I encountered Family Constellations—I tried to forgive the man who assaulted me. I hoped forgiveness could be a means to healing, a premise that was then, as it is now, very au courant in pop psychology, touted by therapists as a balm for an injured soul (not to mention by many religions . . . I do come from a Catholic background, after all!).

How has forgiveness gone for you? Honestly, I had a hard time grappling with forgiveness. It was slippery and hard to pin down. What would I be granting my abuser in forgiving him? I tried forgiveness-adjacent practices that I read about in books or magazines, or that I encountered in spiritually minded activities—exercises like "letting go," "sending love" to my rapist, and "seeing him as the little boy he used to be." No matter what I tried, though, no matter how I strove for forgiveness, I was never at peace. My mind remained an endless loop of racing thoughts. I felt resentment and indigestion in my gut, as if I could not process the incident for good. Above all, I felt trapped and uneasy, like I was playing a role. And in a sense, I was. Forgiveness requires that you inhabit the persona of "the bigger person," someone strong who has the power to bequeath something valuable to someone lesser (even if the action is self-interested).

At its heart, forgiveness is less an action than it is a dynamic, and a power dynamic at that. Forgiveness requires one person to be in the right (the victim) and one person to be in the wrong (the perpetrator). Only the person in the right has the power to forgive the person in the wrong. One person is in power; the other is not. My anxiety and queasiness around forgiveness was intimately tied to this dynamic, though I didn't know that at the time. The discomfort I felt in being "the bigger person"—that sense of being trapped—was because I *was* trapped.

Being wronged makes us right. But holding on to our "rightness" —and the power to forgive that comes with it—only renews our fixation on the harm that has been perpetrated against us. It reenergizes our trauma and keeps us stuck. This is why forgiveness (a moral judgment) is an anathema to consenting to what is (a liberating focus on facts, not narratives). Forgiveness is predicated on blame. When we consent to what is, on the other hand, we suspend moral judgment. Again, this doesn't mean you condone what happened. It means you surrender your narratives about what happened in order to be released from them. When we release blame, *we do not release the perpetrator from blame*. We release *our hold* on the blame. We release ourselves from the dynamic. The perpetrator is still very much responsible for what they have done—but their fate is not our responsibility. This doesn't mean you can't or shouldn't seek justice or speak truth to power, but it does mean you should do so in service to the future (i.e., preventing similar crimes or abuses from happening to others) and with the understanding and agreement that you are not in control of the outcome.

When you release yourself from a system of blame (or its implied counterpart, forgiveness), you respect your fate and the fate of the person who harmed you. Okay, deep breath. This unequivocally does *not* mean you approve of what they've done. *It means you acknowledge and accept that you cannot be responsible for the fate of another.* It means that you do not take on as your responsibility whatever cards that person will be dealt as a result of their actions. You recognize that their fate is outside your domain. When you acknowledge this, you are no longer bound to your perpetrator. You can put down the burden of attempting to carry them with you on the path of your destiny. How much lighter, how much freer will you be when you set down that weight? No longer expending the effort of carrying such a weight, how much more energy will you have to charge forward?

We are each responsible only for ourselves; this is implicit to consenting to reality. Your actions—*your choices*—are your own, just as your perpetrator's actions, stemming from their choices, belong solely to them. We may be caught in entanglements or have rough luck with fate, but we still have free will. That's part of the beauty of doing this work: In requiring you to take responsibility for yourself, it illuminates that you *do* have the agency to do so, that you have choices. It returns the power to you.

One of my clients, a woman in her forties, had been abused by her father throughout her childhood, and her mother, who was abused by him as well, had never intervened. Her mother often implied that the abuse was the daughter's fault, because she had become pregnant with her out of wedlock, which "angered" the father, who then was "forced" into marrying her, which was when the abuse started. Even at 40-something, my client identified and empathized with her mother, believing quite literally that her mother's fate was her responsibility. Even as she blamed her for not protecting her, she felt her mother had had no choice. She wanted to forgive her so she could focus on working through her issues with her father, the perpetrator. In working together, however, we were able to acknowledge not only her father as perpetrator but her mother as well. In consenting to reality and respecting her mother's fate, my client's mantra became "I am not and was not in charge of my mom's decisions. She did have choices, and she chose not to protect me. I have no price to pay for being alive." She did not forgive her; she consented to what is. Recognizing her mother's choices underscored for her that we all have choices, which she found freeing.

The power imbalance inherent to forgiveness also reinforces and perpetuates an entangling victim-perpetrator dynamic for the family system, as well as making it more difficult for you to consent to what is. In a sense, each time a victim and perpetrator interact, they create an energetic bond, becoming a part, however peripheral, of each other's extended family systems via that bond. (If the perpetrator is a family member, he or she loses his or her rights inherent to that role but never loses their place in the system. Remember, if such a person is excluded, leaving a "hole" in the family system, someone else will be drawn to take his or her place, re-creating the dynamic.) Family systems seek order, as we know; the imbalance in a victim-perpetrator dynamic creates disorder.

When you are wedded to your victim-perpetrator dynamic, you will almost always violate the rule of belonging by excluding your perpetrator, creating further disorder in turn. For a system to be in order, everyone in it must be accepted in their place—even the murderer, rapist, or abuser—in order for you to have peace. *But, Marine,* you might be thinking, *how can we accept those who have harmed us?!* I understand if this is the moment when you feel tempted to throw this book across the room! Think of it this way: Peace is another form of *order*—peace is an absence of fighting, an absence of noise. Those we attempt to shut out will only insist more loudly on making their presence known. They want to be heard; they raise their voices. When we acknowledge and accept a missing person, their need is met and they can withdraw their voice. When every member of a system is in their place, we are *at peace*. The system is in order.

Remember, every member of your (extended) family system has a right to belong to it, regardless of what they've done. This doesn't mean you need to warmly embrace (or embrace at all) someone who has harmed you. Again, this is not about forgiveness. It means acknowledging the reality of their presence. In a constellation setting, for example, the victim has to say, "I see you," but not "I forgive you." It's a form of deep respect for what is. It is an acceptance of *your* fate. The perpetrator will carry their guilt, their shame—and it's not your fucking problem, pardon my French. In this approach, *you* will find peace.

I know it is a deeply uncomfortable idea to include a perpetrator in your extended family system. Remind yourself that the right to belong is value-neutral. Think of the family system as a structure, its integrity dependent on each component of its framework. Remove a component, and its integrity becomes compromised. Eventually, serious problems will plague the structure, or it may even suffer collapse. Missing people are like those missing components. When we reinclude them—when everyone is in their rightful place—order is restored. When we are in our rightful places, we are no longer entangled with one another. The bond between victim and perpetrator is broken, with relief.

When you are able to see your perpetrator in their proper place (as part of your extended family system), you are implicitly acknowledging what is: the reality of the perpetrator in your life. The picture of reality is now complete and therefore clearer, empowering you to consent to it fully. After all, it's pretty hard to consent to what is when you can't acknowledge what is. When you are able to acknowledge the perpetrator's place in your extended family system, your attention can shift from their fate to your destiny. To practice doing so, you can visualize your perpetrator far behind you, a speck on the horizon of your past. They are *there*, in their place; you have acknowledged them. You are in your place—and the two are firmly divided.

In my experience, once I was able to see my perpetrator in his rightful place in my extended family system, my ability to consent to what is deepened meaningfully. For 15 years, I fed the bond between my perpetrator and me. Though I toggled between the hypervigilance of being stuck in "on" and the lassitude of being stuck in "off," I consistently experienced revenge fantasies. These were not limited to the punishment I would execute on my rapist—I wanted to hurt and devastate all men. The men on whom I concentrated my rage and distrust (ahem, *all of them*) operated as stand-ins for my perpetrator. A homogenous and undifferentiated mass, they came to function as a screen, in a sense, blurring my ability to see the actual person who had hurt me. In this way, I did not have to look at or acknowledge him directly, which helped keep me "safe."

After acknowledging my perpetrator, including him in his rightful place, and consenting to what is, I understood that I couldn't make anything meaningful of or for myself with revenge or anger. The only thing I could build would be more all-consuming anger and aggression. I didn't want to become a bitter person, brandishing my pain as a weapon in what I had perceived to be the battle of life. I understood that my pain did not define me. It wasn't my identity. It was the product of a situation that had happened long ago, one that, in my case, likely revealed my true purpose.

Consenting to what *is* is difficult, yes, but it is also incredibly brave and profoundly healing. And in healing ourselves—and restoring order to our family system—we engage in an act of generosity and love to those who come after us. We know that the family system will always seek completeness and order. We also know that its primary method for doing so disorders the system further: entanglement.

Victim and perpetrator are twinned energies. When we hold on to victim energy (or perpetrator energy), we fuel an imbalance that disrupts the order of the family system, creating a cycle in which someone in a later generation will be drawn to right the balance, to act for us in an entanglement. In fact, when we commit to despising our perpetrators, we often unwittingly create perpetrators in our children or grandchildren—people who feel justified in their anger as they seek retribution on behalf of those with whom they are entangled. We also perpetuate perpetrator energy through exclusion. As we know, missing people are among the greatest causes of entanglement. A missing family member is a weak point in the structure of the system. The family system will seek to repair that vulnerability by replacing the missing with a member of a subsequent generation, who becomes identified with the excluded person and is drawn into that person's place. Or we may transmit victim energy, creating an entanglement with a child who is compelled to revisit scenarios like the trauma in an attempt to change its outcome. In all of these senses, entanglement is in many ways like a generational trauma response. Whatever has not been taken care of and recognized will happen again. When we acknowledge what is and consent to it, when we include our perpetrators in our family systems, we cut short the cycle of violence and preempt the trauma it creates. This is a remarkable gift we can choose to give our children and our children's children.

Above all, it's a remarkable gift you can give yourself. You cannot forgive the unforgivable. But you can elect to leave your perpetrator to their own fate as you embrace your magnificent destiny. You can relinquish the heavy burden of blame—of responsibility that doesn't belong to you and isn't yours to manage—and, free from its weight, move with a new grace in the direction of your choosing. We all deserve the freedom and the joy of a life that looks forward with hope and rests in the present moment at peace.

AFFIRMATIONS

What happened to me was not my fault.

I make peace with myself.

You stay there, and I stay here.

I am safe.

EXERCISE: Life Flows Forward—Affirming the Future

This is less an exercise than it is a symbolic act dedicated to asserting and affirming the fundamental forward movement and generative energy of life and your ability to connect to and nurture that energy. There are several ways you can choose to do this—all are rooted (pardon the pun) in nature.

- Many cities have community gardens you can join. Not only is this a fantastic way to get your hands dirty and literally ground yourself in the cycles of life, it is also a way to connect to something larger than yourself—your community. This is a fantastic way to practice a systemic worldview.

- Don't want to have to go somewhere else to get your green on? Selecting and caring for a houseplant is a great way to keep a visual reminder of your commitment to healing and growth in your home.

- If you don't have a green thumb, volunteer with an organization that plants trees. This can be a one-time commitment, though you might find it so rewarding that it becomes something you do annually.

- Don't feel you have the time for volunteering? Donate to a charity that will plant a tree in your name, or in the name of one of your ancestors. As you click that "pay now" button, visualize that tree, out in the world, growing and resilient. Wherever you go, wherever you are, that tree will be out there.

Conclusion

Healing Is an Act of Faith

My clients are my heroes. Family Constellations demands a kind of brutal candor with the self. It takes major guts to look at yourself with honesty—to abandon your narratives and *acknowledge what is*—and commit to your healing. Because healing isn't a place we arrive where everything is fine and all our bad feelings go away. No. Healing is a process, a journey: a path you can't walk without confronting your shadows. It takes courage to heal. Even though they hurt, toxic patterns and addictive behaviors feel safe in their familiarity, comfortable. It's so much easier to stay stuck than it is to change and face the unknown. Choosing to set out on a path of healing is a bold act of defiance. It's optimism in the face of fear. It's an act of faith in yourself. It's an embrace of the unknown, of the future. A future *you* get to write.

The healing path of Family Constellations is one of taking ownership of your life. It's healing as an act of supreme agency. Healing is saying, "I am an adult; I am responsible for my life. I'm in charge." Healing is finally knowing what you want and what you don't want—and being willing to do what's necessary to get rid of the latter and bring the former into reality. I think it's pretty badass to be like, *Okay, let me take care of my shit.* It's like you already know you deserve so much better; it's a recognition of your magnificence. It's choosing yourself first. It's choosing hope. Whenever I get a notification that I have a new booking, I already know that person is on their way to something bigger, more beautiful, and more aligned.

And even though chances are you and I haven't met, you're my hero too. The moment you picked up this book, you chose yourself first. You chose hope. Hope for a different, freer, more authentic life.

It's never too late to choose healing. I've been so privileged to witness so many of my clients embark on their journeys, at all stages of life. My client Carrie's embrace of her destiny affected me deeply. Carrie came to me at age 60, after her adult daughter participated in one of my workshops. She said she was curious about the method, though she seemed almost skeptical and like she wasn't quite sure what she was doing in my office. Carrie was the only girl among her four siblings. Her parents were Irish immigrants, and they were deeply devout Catholics and both very stoic. Her father was extremely authoritarian, and her stay-at-home mother did everything for him and Carrie's three brothers, who were like the princelings of the household. Carrie's role was primarily to help her mother take care of the house and its male inhabitants—to listen to the men. After high school, Carrie skipped college and married early, following in her mother's footsteps. She had six kids: two girls and four boys.

When I met Carrie, she and her husband had been married for 35 years. Carrie told me that her relationship with her kids, who were all out of the home by this point, but especially with her daughters, was strained. It made her profoundly unhappy, as she loved them deeply. But they all felt that their father had been too controlling and too severe and that Carrie should have stepped in but never did. Carrie knitted her fingers together as she spoke, looking at her hands. "I didn't feel I had a voice," she said. "I did everything for my children. My husband never helped me. He was the provider. He didn't share his emotions. I feel like I did my best, but I do want to offer something different to my children, specifically my daughters."

Over two years, Carrie bravely worked to make peace with her childhood and her cultural inheritance. It takes guts to break free from something so deeply ingrained. She was able to embrace her feminine essence outside of motherhood and to take a position of authority in relation to her own feelings, to express her real emotions. It was beautiful to witness her take the best of her Irish heritage and her true essence as a woman, to accept her parents and what they had to offer. Her relationship with her daughters changed drastically; they were finally able to talk to each other and connect with emotional intimacy. In a way, it was like Carrie was reconciling with motherhood, an identity she had never felt she had actively chosen, and with womanhood, which she had previously resented for the limitations it imposed on her life. With her daughters, she was discovering how women can come together to build something great. And she finally felt that she had a central role in her family, rather than being subordinate to her husband. As she modeled vulnerability, her relationship with him shifted. Carrie was finally free to be herself: to voice her thoughts and feelings, to experience herself fully as a woman in every dimension. The moment Carrie showed up in my office, she chose healing, she chose hope, she chose freedom.

Healing means freedom. The freedom of creating the life that you truly want based on your own terms, beliefs, and values. Not being afraid of not pleasing everyone, of being rejected or abandoned because you think or feel differently. Healing is self-love. Healing is falling madly in love with your true self, whoever that is. Healing is being safe with yourself, secure with yourself, experiencing belonging in your soul.

We all want to belong. Part of the beauty of Family Constellations is how it shows us how utterly natural, how universal, how human this need is. That's the first thing as a child, as a newborn, that we know we must do—secure our belonging. Our survival depends on it. When we don't belong, we are not seen, we are not heard, we are not recognized. Rejection, exclusion, is erasure of the self. A decade as a therapist has shown me unmistakably that almost all of our issues, our problems, our toxic behaviors go back to belonging.

Unfortunately, sometimes we experience a trauma that severs our sense of belonging, or our parents or caregivers could not or would not see us, hear us, recognize us. (Sometimes, too often, it's both.) Children are crafty; they'll do what it takes to have their needs met. As a child, you'll find other ways to be seen, to be heard, to be recognized—to belong. Maybe your father suffered from depression, so you became a clown. Maybe your mother drank, so you became an enabler, co-dependent. In these ways, you secured your value to others.

And this is where the trickiest, scariest, and bravest part of healing comes into play—when healing feels, perversely, like a threat to your self-worth. On your healing journey, you'll experience real resistance. You probably have already as you've read these pages. These moments of resistance are a sign of progress, though. They underscore the change that's burgeoning within, a change that is frightening because it feels threatening to belonging as we have known it. When we start to relinquish the mechanisms that we've relied on to secure our belonging, so to speak—addiction, disordered eating, compulsive spending, workaholism, abusive relationships—we do risk, or feel we are risking, alienating our loved ones. It can feel like they may no longer accept us. When we choose to restore healthy belonging via love, respect with acceptance, we might wonder whether our family will welcome us belonging in that way. In that moment, it can feel a little like, *Shit, am I still going to move on? Or am I just going to stay stuck here because I'm so afraid that my family will never accept me with my new way of belonging?*

This is totally normal. More than normal! It's pretty common actually. It's okay to be afraid. Remember, everything that you have been doing in terms of healing has been in service to your inner child. It takes bravery to break free from your family's story, from your family system's disorder, and it takes guts to be willing to claim out loud, "Yes, I want to be better; I want to feel better; I want to heal. I want to expand myself; I want to blossom. I want to thrive and to succeed." It takes a lot of courage.

That's why I say that healing is about falling madly in love with yourself. When you love yourself, you choose yourself. In order to really be fully aligned and happy, you need to love yourself. There's no way around it. Of course, when I say you need to love yourself, I don't mean that you'll never experience self-doubt again. It's not like every day you'll be walking around thinking, *Oh my god, I love myself, I love myself, I love myself.* You'll still have your ups and downs; you'll still have your shitty days, *but* you will always find that strength, that courage to go back to your happiness. Faced with a tough decision, you'll choose your highest good. You will always choose yourself because you'll know that by choosing yourself, you'll be equipped to resolve the situation.

My healing journey has been all about choosing to love myself—to heal my relationship to my father, to men, to my body, to my sexuality, to love itself. When I was growing up, my "happily ever after" meant meeting my Prince Charming, getting married, having two or three kids, a big dog, and horses—all by age 30. And, well . . . that's not *quite* how it worked out. I haven't met "the one," and 30 is in the rearview mirror. When I embarked on my Family Constellations journey, I believed I was over that young girl's fantasy. The truth is, I was still caught up in a deep-seated belief that I need a partner to feel loved and desired. Even after so many years of work, I still struggle with it (healing is a journey, after all), but Family Constellations has helped me hold on to the reality that love starts with me. The trauma of being sexually assaulted and raped at 13 cut me off from belonging—belonging to my own body and to myself. I disassociated and numbed out to survive. I was just a kid, but looking back I'm amazed at how strong I was. I can see now how all along I've drawn on that resilience, even during—especially during—some of the most difficult times in my life. I was able to recognize my resilience—to start seeing myself clearly—once I was able to fully acknowledge the trauma itself, to acknowledge what is. That has been one of Family Constellation's greatest gifts to me. Celebrating that resilience has helped me honor myself, to take myself as I am, without apologizing for who I am. I have always felt a pressure to make myself smaller; now I am unapologetically me.

My happiness, your happiness, our happiness, is not about a partner, a certain kind of career, an ideal appearance. No. It's about loving life, knowing life matters, and so your life matters and *you matter*. If you give up on yourself, if you go against your own will, sooner or later whatever uneasiness or difficulty you might have temporarily pushed away or submerged will always resurface. You can't run away from your shadows forever. That's the beauty of this work. When we acknowledge what is, we cast light on our shadows. The shadows vanish, or rather the shame around them vanishes, and they become one of your strengths. It helps to remember that your shadows—your resistance—are, in a way, here to protect you. For me, I had a lot of anger and aggression just below the surface, and they would come out in relationships. I was ashamed and tried harder to suppress them, but they were only defense mechanisms. I was afraid of being hurt, so I struck out first (emotionally). I was protecting myself—you know, *I'll hurt you before you can hurt me*. Behind it was the fear of love. Shining a light on that anger, acknowledging it, opened the way for me to understand it and to harness it. When we choose healing, when we choose to confront our darkness, we let in light; we gain empathy for ourselves and insight into the motivations *behind* our actions. That's the start of change.

Choosing yourself first is never selfish. In fact, I think what's selfish is always putting your shit out on the table, unloading on your friends and family at every brunch, lunch, and dinner. How many people constantly show up as victims, going through the litany of every way they've been wronged? It's exhausting. *That's* selfish. It's easier to complain; it's easier to blame others, to blame your environment. And of course, sometimes I do it too, but I catch myself pretty quickly now. I take responsibility. I stop and ask myself, *What do you want to do? What do you want to create? Stop bullshitting yourself.*

The only thing standing between where you are now and where you would like to be is the bullshit you keep telling yourself, the flow of negative thoughts, of toxic thoughts. There is no room in Family Constellations for bullshit—that's part of what drew me to it so powerfully in the beginning. As facilitators, we learn that just because someone is telling you their story, that doesn't necessarily mean they want to find a resolution. The story might be an excuse, an addiction . . . and nothing else. When someone starts talking about their feelings, emotions, and sensations, that's when we know the person is ready to finally peel off the layers of their shield of protection. It's time to tell those toxic thoughts, that tired old story, *You know what? Thank you so much, but we're done here. I'm choosing me.*

Healing is a reconciliation between your past and present. It's the pure reconciliation of what was and what is. Healing means bringing back together what was once separated. So often, that means people themselves. I know myself better through whatever you're triggering within me; I know myself better through my dynamics with my friends, my co-workers, my boss, my family, my lover, my children. We are all part of each other's healing, no matter what. We are not on our own in healing. When I heal, I offer you my healing. We lead by example, and that's beautiful. We heal together.

Healing is an ongoing, lifelong process, for sure. Yes, it's hard, and yes, it takes courage. But I think it can be fun too. It's fun to know yourself. It's fun to understand yourself, and you should not be afraid of knowing yourself—that's probably one of the most precious investments in your joy you can give yourself. Do the work, but enjoy life along the way. At the end of the day, the work that you will be doing will make sense only if you live your life to the fullest and you go within with fearlessness. Bet on yourself and take risks. You needn't be afraid of starting over again because you will just see it as a new chapter, a next adventure. We have the tendency to overcomplicate things or overthink, but the more I've been working with clients and on myself as well, the more I can see that healing happens through simplicity. When we are honest with ourselves, we vocalize our emotions, take responsibility for the life that we want, consent to what happened, and accept and respect our families as they are. Healing happens when we fall madly in love with who we are.

Everyone deserves to be happy; everyone deserves to heal their wounds. Everyone deserves to be optimistic and hopeful in regard to their future. Have faith in yourself. Have faith that there is always a solution available to you, within yourself. Nothing is stuck as long as you believe in yourself. As my favorite poet, René Char—who was also a member of the French Resistance—wrote, *"Impose ta chance, serre ton bonheur et va vers ton risque. A te regarder, ils s'habitueront"*: "Impose your chance, hold tight to your happiness and go toward your risk. Looking your way, they'll follow."

Reading List

If you'd like to read more about Family Constellations therapy and trauma, here are a few books I recommend:

By Bert Hellinger (Founder of Family Constellations)
Love's Own Truths: Bonding and Balancing in Close Relationships

Love's Hidden Symmetry: What Makes Love Work in Relationships

Looking into the Souls of Children: The Hellinger Pedagogy in Action

No Waves without the Ocean

The Ancestor Syndrome: Transgenerational Psychotherapy and the Hidden Links in the Family Tree, by Anne Ancelin Schützenberger

Family Constellations: A Practical Guide to Uncovering the Origins of Family Conflict, by Joy Manné

It Didn't Start with You: How Inherited Family Trauma Shapes Who We Are and How to End the Cycle, by Mark Wolynn

Endnotes

CHAPTER 3

1. Bert Hellinger, *Looking into the Souls of Children: The Hellinger Pedagogy in Action* (Berchtesgaden, Germany: Hellinger Publications, 2014).

2. Joy Manné, Ph.D., *Family Constellations: A Practical Guide to Uncovering the Origins of Family Conflict* (Berkeley, CA: North Atlantic Books, 2009).

CHAPTER 4

3. Bert Hellinger and Gabriele ten Hövel, *Acknowledging What Is: Conversations with Bert Hellinger* (Phoenix, AZ: Zeig, Tucker & Theisen Inc., 1999).

4. Ibid.

5. Ibid.

Index

A

Abortion, 11

Absent family members
about, 40, 45–46
affirmations, 52
author's personal story, 50–51
blame and, 168–170
client stories, 46–48
defined, 45
exercise, 53
honoring, 48–50
secrets and, 51–52

Abusive relationships, 71, 99–101,
127–128, 144–146, 157, 167

Acceptance
exercise, 19–20
following adoption, 117

Acknowledging what is principle
about, xix, 15–18
affirmations, 18, 162
blame and, 166, 168–169
client stories, 25–28
exercises, 19–20, 163–164
honoring our ancestors through,
18, 21–25
for trauma, 152, 159–164. *See also*
Wholeness, from fragmentation to

Adolescence, 101–102, 116

Adoption, 115–117

Affirmations
for enlightened love, 96, 105, 123
for order and belonging, 18, 52,
57, 96, 123
for origin stories, 18, 37
for parents, 72, 87–88
for romantic relationships, 136,
148
for wholeness, 158, 162, 171

Affirming the future exercise,
171–172

Altars, for honoring ancestors, 38

Ancestors. *See* Honoring our
ancestors

Anne (client), 132–133

Archetypes, 9, 75–76, 80–81, 113

Avoidant strategy, 155

B

Balance, as second order of love, 109

Belonging. *See* Order and belonging

Bert Hellinger Institute, xviii

Berthold, Natalie, xii, xvi

Birthdays, 55

Black Lives Matter, 36

Blame. *See* Releasing blame

Blechner, Michelle, xii, xvi–xvii

Blended families, 112–115

Blind love, 5, 101

Boundaries
about, 106
adoption and, 117
choosing ourselves as, 144–145
enlightened love and, 101–105
exercise for setting, 106–109
for parents, 71, 79, 101–105
for siblings, 122
for stepparents, 113
types of, 106–107

Bowing exercise, 72–73

Brothers and sisters, 10, 116–122, 131–132, 145–146

Bystander training, 14–15

C

Call of ghosts. *See* Absent family members

Carrie (client), 174

Character judgements, 22

Children
life force energy between parents and, 4, 70–71, 72–73, 87–88
loyalty of, 5, 93–95
mindset of, 16, 98–109. *See also* Inner child

Choosing life exercise, 159

Classism, 24–25

Consenting to what is principle
about, 159–161
affirmations, 162
author's personal story, 162
client stories, 161
exercise, 163–164
releasing blame and, 169–170

Constellation exercise, xiii–xiv

Control, 16–17, 18, 20

COVID-19 pandemic, 35–36, 64–65

Croatia, 29–30

Cultures and cultural histories
client stories, 174–175
exercise, 37–38
healing and, 174–175
origin stories and, 22, 24–25, 31, 37–38
parental expectations and, 74–75, 80–81, 110–111
shared names and, 54

D

"Daddy issues," 125–126, 128, 130–132, 134–135

Dead, realm of, 45

Death days, 55

Death, fear of, 46–47

Depression, 156

Destinies, 57

Detaching from outcomes, 20

Disinterested observation, xiii–xiv

Disorder, 4–8, 91–96, 114

Divorce, 11, 111–115, 126–128, 131, 134

Dutch Hunger Winter (1944–45), 6–7

E

Echoing patterns, 53–59, 132–134

Ego, 17–18

EMDR (eye movement desensitization and reprocessing) therapy, xi–xii

Emotions (negative), 19

Enlightened love, 91–124
about, 101, 142
adoption and, 115–117

affirmations, 96, 105, 123
author's personal story, 114–115
blended families and, 112–115
blind love comparison, 101
boundary setting and, 101–105
client stories, 99–101, 103–105,
    116–117, 120–122
disorder and, 91–96
divorce and, 111–115
exercises, 96–98, 106–109,
    123–124
inner child and, 98–109. *See also*
    Inner child
orders of love and, 109–110
precedence and priority for,
    109–124. *See also* Precedence
    and priority
siblings and, 117–122

Entanglements, 39–45
about, 5, 39–41
absent family members as, 40,
    45–52, 53, 168–170
affirmations, 57
author's personal story, 7–8,
    50–51, 56
defined, 5, 39
echoing patterns, 53–57
epigenetics and, 6
exercises, 42–45, 58–59
fate-destiny comparison, 57
honoring our ancestors and,
    20–22
of inner child, 98
with self, as trauma, 151. *See also*
    Wholeness, from fragmenta-
    tion to
shared names, 54–55
signs of, 7, 42–45
suicides and violent deaths,
    49–50
tattoos and, 46

Epigenetics, 6

Everyday interconnectedness, 12,
    14–15

"Everyone has a place" meditation,
    9–11

"Everything happens for a reason,"
    19, 148

Exercises
acknowledging what is principle,
    19–20, 163–164
constellation description, xiii–xiv
for enlightened love, 96–98,
    106–109, 123–124
for entanglements, 42–45, 58–59
for family systems, xiii–xiv,
    12–15, 19–20, 37–38, 42–45,
    53, 55
for inner child, 106–109, 124
for order and belonging, 12–15,
    42–45, 53, 58–59, 96–98,
    123–124
for origin stories, 12–15, 37–38, 55
for receiving and taking, 88–90
for right parents, 72–73, 88–90
for romantic relationships, 136–
    139, 148–149
for wholeness, 159, 163–164,
    171–172

F

Family Constellation Institute, xviii

Family Constellations
author's introduction to, xii,
    xvi–xviii
author's personal transformation,
    xviii–xix
author's professional experiences,
    xviii, xix–xx
basis (foundation) for, xii–xvi
core principles of, xx–xxi, 15–16.
    See also Acknowledging what is
    principle; *Consenting to what is*
    principle
field guide to. *See* Enlightened
    love; Entanglements; Order
    and belonging; Origin stories;
    Parents; Romantic relation-
    ships; Wholeness, from frag-
    mentation to goals of, 7
healing as an act of faith and,
    173–180

overview, xxi–xxiv
power of, xxiv
reading list, 181

Family soul, 4

Family system
about, 1, 3–4
acknowledging what is, 15–20
affirmations, 18, 37
author's personal story, 2, 7–8
entanglements and, 5, 39–45
exercises, xiii–xiv, 12–15, 19–20,
37–38, 42–45, 53, 55
family comparison, 4
generations affected by, 42
intergenerational trauma and, xii
meditation, 9–11
order and, 4–8, 40–41. *See also*
Order and belonging
storytelling and, 1–4. *See also* Origin stories
systems thinking and, 7–8,
12–15, 31

Famine, 6–7

Fate, 20–22, 57, 70, 166, 167

Fathers
acceptance of, 84–85, 87, 95–96
affirmations, 87–88
client stories, 29–30, 67–69,
82–85, 94–96
exercise, 88–90
expectations of, 74, 79–81,
85–86, 87
loyalty to, 93–95
rejection of, 79–85

Favoritism, 118–119

Feminine life force energy, 74–76,
80, 87–88

Forgiveness, 164–166, 167

Fragmentation. *See* Wholeness, from
fragmentation to

G

George (client), 94–96

Germany, 25–28, 31, 33–34

Ghosts. *See* Absent family members

Guadeloupe, 25–28

H

Happiness, xxiv, 15

Healing
as an act of faith, 173–180
from trauma, 151–172. *See also*
Wholeness, from fragmentation to

Hellinger, Bert
on adolescence, 101–102
background, xiv–xv
on happiness, xxiv
legacy of, xviii
on life force energy dynamics, 4
on order and belonging, 94
on parents, 70, 88
on peace, 72
on suffering, 99
on systems thinking, 12

Honoring our ancestors, 20–38
about, 20–21
absent family members, 49–51
acknowledging what is principle
for, 18, 21–25
affirmation, 37
author's personal story, 32–35,
50–51
client stories, 25–30
exercise, 37–38, 55
victim-perpetrator dynamic and,
21–25, 36

Hope, 173–174

Hunger Winter (Netherlands; 1944–
45), 6–7

I

"I am because we are," xiv–xv, 12–15

"I don't know," 42–43

"I hear you," 93, 96–98, 124, 131, 134

"I recognize you," 93, 96–98, 124, 131, 134–135

"I see you," 92–93, 96–98, 124, 131, 134

Immigration narratives, 25–31

In-law relationships, 140–141

Inherited (intergenerational) trauma, xii–xv, 5–6, 40–41. *See also* Entanglements

Inherited Trauma Institute, xviii

Inner child
about, 98–99
adoption struggles and, 117
affirmations for, 105
boundary setting and, 101–105
client stories, 95–96, 98, 99–101, 103–105
exercises, 106–109, 124
healing of, 30, 99, 101–103, 117
of the loyalty, 98–99, 129–131
loyalty of, 98–99, 129–131
meditation, 10–11
romantic relationship issues and, 129
saying yes and, 144–146

Interconnectedness, 4, 7–8, 12–15, 24, 35–36

Interdependence, 4

Intergenerational (inherited) trauma, xii–xv, 5–6, 40–41. *See also* Entanglements

Interrupted movement, 85, 88–90

Intimacy issues, 47–48

Ireland, 25–28

"It did not start with me," 5, 15, 39, 42–45, 54

It Didn't Start With You (Wolynn), xviii

Italy, 31

J

JADE (justify, argue, defend, or explain), 109

Jane (client), 64–66

Jonathan (client), 67–69, 98

Judgment, suspension of, 3, 16–18, 23, 32, 166

K

Key dates and ages, 55–56, 57, 58, 100–101

"Know your place," 119–120

L

Leslie (client), 99–101

Life flows forward exercise, 171–172

Life force energy
conception and, 74
family system dynamics affecting, 4
feminine, 74–76, 80, 87–88
flow of, 8
masculine, 74–75, 80–81, 88
between parents and children, 4, 70–71, 72–73, 87–88
suspended moral judgement and, 16

Lila (client), 128–129

Love
orders of, 96–98, 109–110
relationships and. *See* Enlightened love; Parents; Romantic relationships; Siblings

Loving mirror exercise, 159

Loyalty
  as blind love, 5, 101
  of children, 5, 93–95
  of the inner child, 98–99,
    129–131
  stepparent relationships and, 113

M

Manné, Joy, 71

Mary (client), 25–28

Masculine life force energy, 74–75,
  80–81, 88

Meditations, 9–11, 123–124

Michael (client), 116–117

Miscarriages, 11, 46, 55, 89, 133

Missing people. *See* Absent family
  members

Moral judgment, suspension of, 3,
  16–18, 23, 32, 166

Mothers
  acceptance of, 79, 86–87, 95,
    100–101
  affirmations, 87–88
  author's personal story, 86–87
  client stories, 76–79, 82–85
  exercise, 88–90
  expectations of, 74–75, 85–87
  idealization of, 82–84, 86–87
  rejection of, 74–79, 85, 145–146

N

Names, shared, 54–55, 57, 132–133

Narratives
  of family systems, 1–38. *See also*
    Origin stories
  of parents, 62–64, 66, 69–70
  reframing exercise, 163–164

Nature, 13

Nazism, xiv, 6–7, 26–28

Negative emotions, 19

Netherlands, 6–7

Networked way of seeing, 7–8,
  12–15, 31

New perspectives, new stories exercise, 163–164

"No" is a complete sentence,
  108–109

Norway, 31

Nurturing belonging exercise, 96–98

O

Objectivity. *See Acknowledging what
  is* principle

Order and belonging, 45–59
  about, 4–5, 39–41, 109
  about echoing patterns, 53–57
  absent family members, 40,
    45–52, 53, 168–170
  affirmations, 18, 52, 57, 96, 123
  author's personal story, 50–51,
    56–57
  client stories, 46–48, 94–96
  disorder, 4–8, 91–96, 114
  echoing patterns, 53–57, 132–134
  entanglements and, 53–57
  exercises, 12–15, 42–45, 53,
    58–59, 96–98, 123–124
  in family systems, 23, 40
  honoring our ancestors and,
    48–50
  for the inner child, 98–109. *See
    also* Inner child
  meditation for, 9–11, 123–124
  origin stories and, 4–8
  as parental responsibility, 92–96
  restoration of order, 7
  secrets and, 51–52

Orders of love, 96–98, 109–110

Origin stories, 1–38

about, 1–2
acknowledging what is, 15–20.
    See also Acknowledging what is
    principle
affirmations, 18, 37
author's personal story, 2, 7–8,
    32–35
client stories, 25–30
cultures and cultural histories,
    31, 37–38
exercises, 12–15, 37–38, 55
family system and, 1–15. *See also*
    Family system
honoring, 20–38. *See also* Honor-
    ing our ancestors
"I don't know" as, 42–43
immigration narratives, 25–31
meditation, 9–11
order and, 4–8
religious traditions and, 13–14,
    31–32
traditional therapy-Family Con-
    stellation comparison, 2–4
victim-perpetrator dynamic and,
    21–25, 36

Outcomes, detaching from, 20

Overcoming resistance exercise,
    19–20

P

Parents. *See also* Inner child
    acceptance of, 73–74, 79, 84–87,
        95–96, 100–101
    adoption and, 115–117
    affirmations, 72, 87–88
    author's personal story, 86–87
    boundaries for, 71, 79, 101–105
    client stories, 64–69, 76–79,
        82–85, 94–96, 99–101,
        103–105
    "daddy issues" affecting romantic
        relationships, 125–126, 128,
        130–132, 134–135
    exercises, 72–73, 88–90

    expectations of, 69–70, 74–75,
        79–81, 85–87
    idealization of, 82–84, 86–87
    life energy force between children
        and, 4, 70–71, 72–73, 87–88
    narratives, 62–64, 66, 69–70
    precedence and priorities for,
        110–112
    rejection by, 93–94
    rejection of, 74–85, 145–146
    responsibilities of, 66, 71, 92–96,
        98
    right parents acknowledgement,
        70–71
    sibling relationships and,
        118–119
    stepparents, 10, 112–115
    traditional therapy-Family Con-
        stellation comparison on,
        61–62

Past, erasing or revisiting, 152

Pattern sorting exercise, 58–59

Patterns, echoing, 53–59, 132–134

Personal inventory exercise, 58–59

Phenomenology, xiv–xv

Pierre (client), 82–85

PIM3 gene, 6–7

Precedence and priority, 109–124
    about, 5, 109–111
    adoption and, 115–117
    affirmation, 123
    author's personal story, 114–115
    blended families and, 112–115
    client stories, 116–117, 120–122
    divorces and, 111–112
    exercise, 123–124
    siblings and, 117–122

Prussia, 33–34

R

Rachel (client), 103–105

Racism, 22, 24–25, 36

Rape, xviii–xix, 151–153, 165, 169, 177

Reaching-out movement, 85

Recognition ceremony, 53

Reframing narratives exercise, 163–164

Rejection
as defense mechanism, 105
disorder and, 91–94
fear of, 89, 106
idealization as form of, 82–83
by parents, 93–94
of parents, 74–85, 145–146

Relationship inventory exercise, 136–139, 148–149

Relationships. *See* Enlightened love; Inner child; Parents; Romantic relationships; Siblings

Releasing blame
about, 164, 166–167, 170–171
affirmations for, 171
author's personal story, 165, 169
client story, 167
consenting to what is principle and, 169–170
exercise, 171–172
forgiveness comparison, 164–166, 167
victim-perpetrator dynamic, 165–170

Religious traditions, 13–14, 31–32

Remarriage and repartnership, 112–115

René (client's husband), 132–133

Resistance, overcoming, 19–20, 176

Respect for family members. *See* Honoring our ancestors

Respecting shared stories exercise, 148–149

Right parents, 70–71

Rights, 107–108

Roberto (client), 120–122

Romantic relationships, 125–149
abusive relationships, 99–101, 127–128, 144–146
affirmations, 136, 148
author's personal story, 32–35, 126–128, 130, 145–146
client stories, 128–129, 131–134
ending relationships and, 141–144
exercises, 136–139, 148–149
family system dynamics affecting, 125–126, 128, 130–132, 134–135
immigration origin stories and, 29–30
meditation for, 11
responsibilities and, 146–147
saying yes to, 139–149. *See also* Saying yes to romantic relationships

Ruiz, Don Miguel, 67

S

Saying yes to romantic relationships, 139–149
about, 139–141
affirmations, 148
author's personal story, 145–146
ending relationships and, 141–144
to enlightened love, 142
exercise, 148–149
responsibilities, 146–147

Secret stories, 50–52

Secrets, about absent family members, 51–52

Self-harming behavior, 156

Self-love, 90, 144–145, 175, 177–180

Self-medication, 156

Setting boundaries exercise, 106–109

Sexual assaults, xviii–xix, 151–153, 165, 169, 177

Shared birthdays or death days, 55

Shared dates and ages, 55–56, 57, 58, 100–101

Shared names, 54–55, 57, 132–133

Shared story respect exercise, 148–149

Siblings, 10, 116–122, 131–132, 145–146

Silence, as survival strategy, 155–156

Single parents, 111

Sisters and brothers, 10, 116–122, 131–132, 145–146

Spirituality, 13–14, 31–32

Stepfamily relationships, 10, 112–115

Storytelling. See Narratives

Subjectivity, 17–18

Suffering, 99

Suicides, 44, 46, 49–50, 55

Supportive parents, 103–105

Survival strategies, 154–158

Suspended moral judgment, 3, 16–18, 23, 32, 166

Systems. See Family system

Systems thinking, 7–8, 12–15, 31

T

Take a bow exercise, 72–73

Talk therapy, 2–4, 17, 61–62

Tattoos, 46

The Four Agreements (Ruiz), 67

Therapy. See EMDR therapy; Family Constellations; Traditional therapy

Traditional therapy, 2–4, 17, 61–62

Transcendence, 14

Trauma
defined, 151
disorder and, 5
as fact of life, 162
healing, 151–172. See also Wholeness, from fragmentation to
inherited, xii–xv, 5–6, 40–41. See also Entanglements
survival strategies for, 154–158

Tristan (client), 29–30

Tucker, Suzi, xviii, 5, 112

Tutu, Desmond, 12

U

Ubuntu, xiv–xv, 12–15

V

Values, 107–108

Victim-perpetrator dynamic
acknowledging what is principle for, 25–28
healing and, 165–170
honoring our ancestors and, 21–25, 36

Victor (client's brother), 120–122

Violent deaths, 49–50

Vivienne (client), 76–79

Voltaire, 57

Volunteerism, 14

W

Walking, 13

Wholeness, from fragmentation to,
151–172
about, 151–152
acknowledging what is principle
for, 152, 159–164
affirmations, 158, 162, 171
author's personal story, 152–154,
161, 162, 165, 169, 177–178
client stories, 156–157, 161, 167
consenting to what is principle and,
159–162, 169–170
exercises, 159, 163–164, 171–172
forgiveness comparison, 164–166,
167
releasing blame, 164, 166–167,
169–171
survival strategies, 154–158
victim-perpetrator dynamic,
165–170

Wolynn, Mark, xviii

World War II era, 6–7, 26–28, 33–34

Writing prompts, 162, 163–164

X

Xenophobia, 24–25, 36

Y

Yes. *See* Saying yes to romantic
relationships

Z

Zeig, Tucker & Theisen, Publishers,
xviii

Zulu peoples and culture, xiv, 12

Acknowledgments

As you know, I'm a French woman and English is not my native language. So, first, I want to acknowledge my fabulous team that helped me to give birth to this dream, my book.

Libby—You're not only "my right arm," but you are also the one who completely got me! Thank you so much for our long conversations about Family Constellations and life. Thank you for finding the right words in order to share my passion about Family Constellations.

Coleen—my agent. Thank you for having my back when I was feeling too emotional. And, above all, thank you for trusting me.

Melody—Thank you for your "YES" of being my editor with Hay House. It has been a great adventure to work together.

And Hay House . . . Wooooooow. A dream came true! You were at the top of my list of dream publishers. Thank you for trusting my work. I'm so honored to be your first female French author.

And, last but not least . . . thank you to my family, my friends, my clients, all of you who made a huge difference in my life with one word, one moment, one walk, one dance . . . You know that I have an extraordinary memory (LOL)—I'll never forget your support, help, and unfailing love.

To my mother, the woman of my life, my foundation, my rock, my "mamounette," without you I would not be on Earth(!). You did not give me life just once; you have given me life several times over: the strength to keep going in my darkest moments. Thank you for your unbreakable Love.

To my father, because of whom my Family Constellations journey began—I wanted to understand you so much. Thank you for our father-daughter moments, especially those nights you'd tell me bedtime stories; they are forever in my heart. Thank you for having the courage to come back into my life (and of course Mom's and Titou's lives) after years apart.

To my brother, for always speaking your truth and pushing me beyond my limits. You know how much I love you and I know how much it bothers you, but at the end, like you said: "Even though I don't show it to you, I love you, my sister." Thank you, my little Titou.

To my grandparents, for their protection.

To my aunts, uncles, and cousins, for their love.

And, to the family that I've been choosing for the past 20 years . . . Our friendship is one of my most precious treasures. I love you all so much—Laetitia, Celine, Elodie, Leslie, Priscilla, Laurence, Pierre, my two Estelles, my three Claires, Victoria, Jessica, my two Megans, Denise, Marie, Maeva, Cecilia, Come, Gabrielle, and Jenny. From the bottom of my heart, thank you for your unconditional support and Love. We'll die together!

To my fabulous village of healers, Samantha, Melanie, Kirsten, Susana, Amy, Georgette, Ben, Nina, Emmanuelle, Mimi, Julia, Ludovic, Lily, and Stephanie. Thank you for taking care of me and teaching me how to lean on all of you!

To my teachers, Suzi Tucker and Mark Wolynn.

To my clients, ten years together . . . You are my heroes. Thank you for your trust and sharing your story with me. Every time I share a session with you is an honor.

And to Medhi. My best friend, the second man of my life, as you used to call yourself. Your violent departure opened a wound that I was not sure I could heal from, but, slowly and surely, you showed me the path to reconnect with love and to finally open my heart in order to receive the love from the man that I was dreaming of. Thank you for placing him on my path. I love you.

Finally, to you, my readers. This is a story of a little girl who was highly sensitive. It's a story of a teenager who lost her naivete at the age of 13. It's a story of a young woman who lost her primary foundation at the age of 22 because of her parents' divorce.

It's a story of a young woman who felt abandoned and rejected by her father because he could not cope with the divorce. It's a story of a young woman who thought she found love in the arms of her first husband but was eaten up by jealousy and violence. It's a story of a woman who always felt that she was going to live abroad and have an extraordinary and unpredictable destiny. It's a story of a woman who does not play by the rules but creates her own rules.

It's me. It's you. It's us.

I wrote this book for all those little girls and boys who always had a bigger vision, a bigger dream, that, as crazy as it may have sounded to everyone else, they always believed in. I'm begging you to never apologize for being "too much," I'm begging you to never settle for less than you want, I'm begging you to always prioritize your own happiness before someone else's, and I urge you to fall madly in love with your story. You have the power to create your destiny; do not be afraid of following and trusting your inner voice.

May this book be a lighthouse, a hopeful message that you are not broken and you just need to surrender to what is; this is only where True Love exists.

With all my love,

Marine Sélénée

About the Author

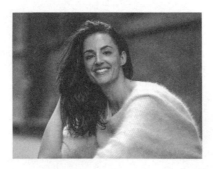

Marine Sélénée is a New York/Miami–based Family Constellations therapist, author and speaker. She offers in-person and virtual private sessions and workshops. She also speaks on panel discussions and at conferences delivering motivational speeches. Her unique approach to Family Constellations helps people heal from family wounds and find individual blocks rooted in the family system. Her clients are able to get to the root of their pain, in order to heal not only themselves but also the generations before and after them. Her greatest passion is sharing the transformative power of Family Constellations.

To learn more about Marine and Family Constellations, visit: **www.marineselenee.com**

Hay House Titles of Related Interest

YOU CAN HEAL YOUR LIFE, the movie,
starring Louise Hay & Friends
(available as a 1-DVD program, an expanded 2-DVD set,
and an online streaming video)
Learn more at www.hayhouse.com/louise-movie

THE SHIFT, the movie,
starring Dr. Wayne W. Dyer
(available as a 1-DVD program, an expanded 2-DVD set,
and an online streaming video)
Learn more at www.hayhouse.com/the-shift-movie

*BLISS BRAIN: The Neuroscience of Remodeling Your Brain
for Resilience, Creativity, and Joy*, by Dawson Church

*HEALING IS THE NEW HIGH: A Guide to Overcoming
Emotional Turmoil and Finding Freedom*, by Vex King

*HEALING YOUR FAMILY HISTORY: 5 Steps to Break Free
of Destructive Patterns*, by Rebecca Linder Hintze

MAMA RISING: Discovering the New You Through Motherhood,
by Amy Taylor-Kabbaz

TRAUMA: Healing Your Past to Find Freedom Now,
by Pedram Shojai, O.M.D., and Nick Polizzi

All of the above are available at www.hayhouse.co.uk

Listen. Learn. Transform.

Listen to the audio version
of this book for FREE!

Gain access to endless wisdom, inspiration, and encouragement from world-renowned authors and teachers—guiding and uplifting you as you go about your day. With the *Hay House Unlimited* Audio app, you can learn and grow in a way that fits your lifestyle . . . and your daily schedule.

With your membership, you can:

- Let go of old patterns, step into your purpose, live a more balanced life, and feel excited again.

- Explore thousands of audiobooks, meditations, immersive learning programs, podcasts, and more.

- Access exclusive audios you won't find anywhere else.

- Experience completely unlimited listening. No credits. No limits. No kidding.

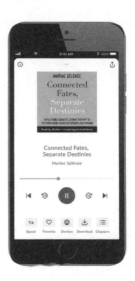

Try for FREE!

Visit **hayhouse.com/audioapp** to start your free trial and get one step closer to living your best life.

Hay House Podcasts
Bring Fresh, Free Inspiration Each Week!

Hay House proudly offers a selection of life-changing audio content via our most popular podcasts!

Hay House Meditations Podcast

Features your favorite Hay House authors guiding you through meditations designed to help you relax and rejuvenate. Take their words into your soul and cruise through the week!

Dr. Wayne W. Dyer Podcast

Discover the timeless wisdom of Dr. Wayne W. Dyer, world-renowned spiritual teacher and affectionately known as "the father of motivation." Each week brings some of the best selections from the 10-year span of Dr. Dyer's talk show on Hay House Radio.

Hay House Podcast

Enjoy a selection of insightful and inspiring lectures from Hay House Live events, listen to some of the best moments from previous Hay House Radio episodes, and tune in for exclusive interviews and behind-the-scenes audio segments featuring leading experts in the fields of alternative health, self-development, intuitive medicine, success, and more! Get motivated to live your best life possible by subscribing to the free Hay House Podcast.

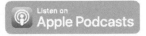

Find Hay House podcasts on iTunes, or visit
www.HayHouse.com/podcasts for more info.

HAY HOUSE

Look within

Join the conversation about latest products, events, exclusive offers and more.

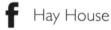 Hay House

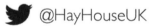 @HayHouseUK

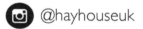 @hayhouseuk

We'd love to hear from you!